Endorsements fo

"All I can say about *Getting Into Your Pants* is well-done. With its down-to-earth tone and conversational writing style, it's a fun and easy read. Better yet, 10+10 is a nutritionally sound, common sense program with three simple rules. Just follow the rules, and you will lose weight while improving your health."

—**Alan Goldhamer, D.C., co-author of** *The Pleasure Trap*

"Follow Dr. Leslie's 10+10 for Life® and all those frustrations from those restrictive diets that never worked will disappear, right along with that weight. Refreshingly, Dr. Leslie masterfully cuts through the confusion and offers a simple solution for losing weight – the right way. And big bonus: she's right on with her food facts. Instead of listening to the food industries' slick marketing ads masquerading as nutrition information, take it from an intelligent, experienced woman who knows her stuff. But even better, she walks her talk. Dr. Leslie is a shining example of glowing health and vibrancy."

—**George Eisman, Registered Dietician, author of** *The Most Noble Diet* **and** *Don't Let Your Diet Add to Your Cancer Risk*

"Dr. Van Romer shares her powerful formula for permanent weight loss and optimal health. *Getting Into Your Pants* is a book that will motivate and inspire people to make positive changes in their health and their life."

—**Joel Fuhrman, M.D., author of** *Eat To Live* **and** *Eat For Health*

"Dr. Van Romer's book, *Getting into Your Pants*, extends the amazing broad-based effects of a plant-based diet to that all-important need - losing weight and keeping it off. I highly recommend it."

—**T. Colin Campbell, Ph.D., author of** *The China Study* **and Jacob Gould Schurman Professor Emeritus of Nutritional Biochemistry at Cornell University**

"*Getting Into Your Pants* is an entertaining read and a great review of the ten thousand reasons you need to follow a low-fat vegan diet."

—**John McDougall, M.D., author of** *The McDougall Program – Twelve Days to Dynamic Health* **and** *The McDougall Program for a Healthy Heart*

Getting

into

Your

Pants

Published by Advantage, Charleston, South Carolina.
Member of Advantage Media Group.

ADVANTAGE is a registered trademark and the Advantage colophon is a trademark of Advantage Media Group, Inc.

Printed in the United States of America.

ISBN: 978-1-59932-072-4
LCCN: 2008921746

Most Advantage Media Group titles are available at special quantity discounts for bulk purchases for sales promotions, premiums, fundraising, and educational use. Special versions or book excerpts can also be created to fit specific needs.

For more information, please write: Special Markets, Advantage Media Group, P.O. Box 272, Charleston, SC 29402 or call 1.866.775.1696.

Getting
into
Your
Pants

Add 10 +10 for Life®!

Dr. Leslie Van Romer

Illustrations by Scott Diggs Underwood

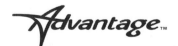

To my father and mother, Ed and Marilyn Van Romer,
who gave me the roots to grow and the wings to soar.

Warning: Disclaimer

The information in this book is not intended to diagnose or treat any condition or disease or to substitute for competent medical advice for your specific problems. If you are taking medications or experiencing any health problems, including but not limited to type 1 and type 2 diabetes, consult your health care practitioner before making dietary changes. If transitioning to weight-loss, health-supporting, and disease-fighting eating habits is safe for you, ask your practitioner to partner with you by monitoring your progress with routine check-ups and blood work.

Contents

Acknowledgements
With Love and Gratitude

We are all human beings residing on the same planet. Whether we know each other or not, we are intricately and inextricably intertwined with one another. Therefore, we are all equally responsible for the creation of this book. The message within is not mine. It is a universal message that has been told but must be told again and again – until we get it. It is a plea to open minds and hearts, raising the level of awareness and thus the quality of life – your life and others around the globe. I am merely a messenger.

First and foremost, I thank you. Messages are meaningless unless there is someone willing to listen, really pay attention, and then transform words and ideas into actions. Here you are – stepping into the food and weight arena one more time, in spite of old wounds and deep scars. Your courage and sheer guts are truly inspirational. You touch my heart. This time, may victory be yours by shedding your armor and layers, leaving you feeling good about the unique and beautiful person you are, filled with wonder, purpose, joy, peace, and kid-like fun.

Second, I kiss the feet of my editors, Liz Blazey and Wendy Dunster – yes, it took two of them to corral this wild filly, as she bucked, kicked, and nipped with every written word. If you find my writing clear and concise, it is largely because of their intelligence, expertise, insights, and finesse with the snap of their whip and softness of touch.

Wendy Dunster plays more than the role of editor in my life. As my big sister and friend, she is my angel on earth. She fully embraces me and, more significantly, my life's mission. She knows how important this message is and works tirelessly to assist me in relaying that message. While I wrote and rewrote, she dried my tears of frustration and lightened my moments of doubt and darkness more times than I care to admit.

Katy Nichols and Diane Williamson, my teammates and dear friends, prodded and pulled this book out of me. Their daily mantra "you've gotta write a book" gave me no wiggle room, if I cherished my peace. For twenty and fifteen years respectively, their hard work, bull-dogged loyalty, and rock-solid confidence in my potential catapulted me over every hurdle toward our shared goals. My vision became theirs. Our synergy fueled the evolvement of our vision and the tenacity to pursue it – the three of us together.

Jeannette Cullison, my first mentor and now deceased, believed in me before I knew there was something within me to believe in. Her wisdom, connection with the spirit dimension, and unwavering certainty gave me the impetus I needed to open doors of self- and other-awareness and step through those doors one by one. Helen Korn, my second mentor and also deceased, emphasized and reinforced every one of Jeanette's lessons. I am indebted to these two dear sages for guiding me to my path. Although I know they are watching over me, I miss them both terribly.

I am deeply grateful to my former husband and still my champion, J.M. Kuno, who continues to love and support me for exactly who I am and understands how my work is my world. His generosity of spirit and bigness of heart exemplify that one can always give more.

And where would all of us be without the visionary pioneers – those rare and bold individuals who not only see the truth but align their lives in accordance with the truth. Furthermore, they honor their gift and responsibility of clear vision by dedicating their lives to opening eyes and uplifting lives around the globe. You warriors know who you are, even if I don't mention your name. My humble gratitude to you and to Dr. John and Mary McDougall, John Robbins, Dr. T. Colin Campbell, Dr. Neal Barnard, Dr. Joel Fuhrman, Dr. Caldwell Esselstyn, Dr. Alan Goldhamer, Dr. Douglas Lisle, Dr. Susan Smith Jones, Brenda Davis, Vesanto Melina, Harvey and Marilyn Diamond, Dr. Frank Sabatino, Jack LaLanne, George Eisman, and all the grand pioneers, like Dr. B.J. Palmer, N.W. Walker, and Herbert Shelton, who left their legacies. And a special thank you to all support individuals and teams.

Many hugs and kudos to my dear patients. I treasure their gracious gift: sharing themselves. Our mutual trust, respect, and genuine caring have built my knowledge, warmed my heart, and fed my soul for almost thirty years, spurring my personal growth and insights into how they feel and think, and what really matters to them.

All people and life experiences prepared and positioned me to be introduced to Dr. Tony Palermo, my mentor, coach, and friend. His brilliance, talents, uncanny sense of people, and belief in me helped me laser through the layers, removing blocks that interfered with my ability to tap into my core and pools of potential. Assisted by his strong, gentle guiding hand, I stepped through the doorway to freedom – the freedom to be me and to transform my vision into reality. Creativity, inner peace, and self-perpetuating exhilaration resulted from that freedom to just be.

My children, Rafael, Erin, and Nika, the loves of my life, taught me the most life-impacting lessons of all: to love without condition and to honor individuals, without judgment and expectation, for whom they are. It is true that all human beings and their paths are equally important to the thriving matrix of human kind.

Foreword
By Narinder Duggal, B.Sc.(Pharm), M.D., CGP, BCPP, FRCPC, FASCP

As the medical director of Liberty Bay Internal Medicine in Poulsbo, Washington, and specialist in internal medicine, pharmacology, diabetes, hypertension, and blood lipids, I have witnessed my patients' medications increase, right along with their weight. No matter how much I emphasized the life-threatening danger of extra weight, the weight still clung to them. The unfortunate consequences: their health was compromised, their hope floundered, and I was frustrated. I tried working with several nutrition experts, but they produced the same disappointing results that I did – no results when it came to motivating people to lose weight.

Then the opportunity presented itself to team up with Dr. Leslie Van Romer. Dr. Van Romer spun her magic, and impressively, my patients lost weight. Quite frankly, I was shocked, and humbled. My patients were beyond thrilled and so was I. Fortunately for all of us, whether struggling with weight or just trying to eat better, she spins that same magic in *Getting Into Your Pants*.

Getting Into Your Pants is very valuable for its easy-to-follow eating program, 10+10 for Life®. But more than that, this book captures Dr. Leslie's essence – her down-to-earth nature, her infectious joy for living, and her genuine love for people – and is an ***extraordinary must-read*** for everyone with the desire to live longer and better.

Of all the lessons that Dr. Van Romer has taught me, one stands above all the rest. Healing and self-evolving do not come from a diagnosis, a pill, or a technically brilliant procedure. They come from the innate power of the human body, the resilience of the human spirit, universal and self-love, and from human connection. I am grateful to call Leslie my colleague, my mentor, and my friend. And you will soon understand why.

Introduction

"But, Mooooom, I Hate Those Pants"

The phone rings.

It's my daughter. Her name is Nika.

I know instantly. She is frustrated – to the point-of-tears frustrated.

In spite of my growling stomach, I put aside the salad that I had just made for myself. I know Nika needs all of my attention.

I settle myself down. For once, I just listen. It is hard for me to do sometimes – just listen.

Nika told me she had weighed herself a few days before. Her weight had hit an all-time high. She had sobbed when she saw the number on the scale. Now, sobbing over the phone, she felt ashamed and weak, embarrassed and lazy. She felt isolated – all alone in her agony; she was desperate.

It had taken several days to get up the nerve to tell her husband how much she weighed – a courageous act in itself, if you ask me. Some things are just too personal and private to share – even with, or especially with, husbands.

Her clothes are too tight. She's been sick every month with a cold or flu. She's tired most of the time, and she is tired of being tired. She is only 24-years-old; she is young, but she feels old.

She hates her weight. She hates her body. And she hates not feeling good about herself.

"The worst part," she says, "is that I've cut way down on my portions, and I exercise hard every day and have for a long time. But I still can't lose weight. In fact, my weight keeps creeping up. I just don't get it."

Her next words break my heart.

"I am fat, and I hate myself like that."

Her pain is my pain – there is no separation.

I can't help it – tears slide silently down my cheeks. Still wordless, I wait for direction from my wounded child.

Then Nika boldly opens the gate and steps into the minefield of a delicate self-esteem.

"Can you help me?" she asks.

She is quiet – perfectly quiet – waiting for my response.

Knowing I could crush her with a word, I collect myself.

My thoughts flashed back to that moment when I had forced Nika, then 8-years-old, to wear bright, pink, polyester pants with an elastic waistband and a matching top. Her pudgy tummy ruled out the option for regular jeans. I happened to think the pink pants were cute. She didn't. In fact, she had hated those pants. None of her friends wore them. She cried and cried, humiliated by those "fat pants." Her tears devastated me and the thought of those tears still sting to this day.

I quickly scan my mind for any inklings of wisdom tucked away from years of guiding women (and a fair share of men) with weight woes, most of whom felt just like Nika – confused, frustrated, alone, and helpless without hope.

I take a deep breath and gently tiptoe into Nika's trust and confidence by asking her a couple of telltale questions.

"First, Nika, do you really, really want to lose weight?"

Without hesitation, she says, "Yes, Mom, I do; I really want this. I'm sick of this weight."

I can tell she means it.

"Second, why do you want to lose weight?"

"I'm doing this for me," she says. "I just want to feel good about myself."

I know she is ready. I know that she has reached that intangible tipping point, spurring her to make an unbreachable commitment to herself.

And then I say to her, "If you will tell me honestly exactly what you eat, listen with an open mind to what I have to say, and follow through what we, together, design for you, I promise you will lose noticeable weight within a month. Not only that, you will reach a reasonable weight loss goal within a year."

I don't make promises unless I can keep them – especially to vulnerable young women, and especially to my own children.

Nika and I spend the next hour tailor-making an eating plan doable for her.

By the end of our time together, Nika's tears and frustration disappear, replaced by genuine excitement and hope – hope that she can and will get down to the pants she longs to wear.

Three Weeks Later...

It's a hectic morning in my office. I'm with patients. My assistant, Katy, comes back and tells me that there's someone on the phone I need to talk to – right then. After twenty years of working with Katy, when Katy tells me to jump, I jump – simple.

It's my daughter, Nika. She apologizes for pulling me away from patients. She knows I'm busy. She just couldn't wait one minute longer to talk to me. She's absolutely flying high.

"Guess what, Mom?" she rattles off to me. "In three weeks, I've lost 15 pounds!" She's ecstatic.

She fits into pants the next size down. Her other clothes are loose on her. Her upcoming graduation outfit had to be altered down – twice. She feels energized and better about herself than she has in years.

I ask her whether she feels deprived or hungry. "No, not at all," she says, "I just do what you said. I fill up on the right foods – like lots of fruits, salads, and vegetables. I eat until I'm full and satisfied. I still eat meat sometimes, but I got rid of cheese, butter, oils, and snacks before bed."

Then Nika confides in me a stinging revelation that she had never told anyone – not her husband, not her best friend, and especially not me. She had always thought the only way she could lose weight was by starving herself or by getting sick. She says that had been her experience in the past.

"But I have found out for myself," she continues, "that losing weight is not about eating or not eating; it's about what you eat. And for the first time in my life, I feel like I am in control of my body, and I feel wonderful! I actually look forward to eating fruit and salads now."

Nika says that before the weight came off, she wanted people to notice her and compliment her on how she looked, just because she had worked so hard with her daily exercise. She wanted and needed the strokes from folks to feel good about herself.

"But now," she says, "I feel so good about myself that, all of a sudden, I don't care anymore what people think or say. In fact, if they ask me if I'm on a diet, I just say 'no' because I'm not, and I change the subject."

As I hang up the phone and return to my waiting patients, my heart sings to the tune of the song in Nika's heart.

25 POUNDS DOWN, SPIRITS SOAR

Three Months Later...

It was another busy Friday morning in the office. My gracious patients are waiting patiently for their time with me. Katy comes back. "A phone call for you, Dr. Leslie."

It's Nika again. Her excitement is electrifying. She has just hopped off the scale. In three months, she has lost 25 pounds. She has just gotten into guess what? Those coveted pants – a size 6 no less. Wow – a size 6 pants! She can hardly believe it. She's lighter than she's been in years.

The best part – people are asking her to help them lose weight just like she's doing. She's thrilled with herself and even more thrilled that she can now lead other people by example.

Nika has accomplished her goal. She feels great about herself and how she looks. She sounds like a different person than that desperate girl three short months before.

Tears spontaneously spring to my eyes. My youngest daughter, haunted for years by that lingering nightmare of extra rolls and bright, pink pants, is finally happy – from the inside out.

MOTHERS, DAUGHTERS, AND PANTS

Of my three children, it's Nika whom I've watched struggle most of her life with her weight, her bad feelings about her self-perceived "ugly" body, and her self-esteem. It took twenty-four years for her to be mature enough, secure enough, and courageous enough to ask her own mother for help; her mother whose passion just happens to be guiding others to achieve weight, self, and health goals.

It took me twenty-four years to be mature enough, secure enough, and open enough to reply without judgment and preaching.

When Nika called, I was honored and humbled by her request. As all of us moms know, mother-daughter relationships can be very delicate. It's an art for a mother to know when to be quiet and when to offer advice.

I don't claim to have mastered that art – not by a long shot, as both my daughters (and son) would freely tell you. However, I have learned that offering unsolicited advice about weight is taboo in the world of mothers and daughters. My daughter's brave plea for help not only catalyzed her freedom from her padded prison, but opened that locked door into a deeper level of our mutual trust, acceptance, and love – a precious lifetime gift for both of us.

MY DAUGHTER, MY TEACHER

Witnessing Nika's struggle with weight gave me another gift – awareness of the heartbreaking devastation, on many levels, which extra fat can cause. You see, I'm often asked whether I, myself, have struggled with weight. If not, how would I know how it feels to be a weary warrior in that constant battle? That's a fair question and deserves a straightforward, honest answer.

The simple answer: no, I haven't struggled with weight. However, that doesn't mean I wouldn't be caught in that sticky weight web today if I hadn't changed my habits early in my life. Thirty-five years ago I tipped the scale thirty pounds heavier than I do today. But because I was fortunate enough to start my journey to my ideal weight and level of health with better eating and exercise habits while still in my twenties, those thirty pounds gradually, naturally slipped away and stayed away – just like they can for you.

Even though I attained my ideal weight fairly easily, my baby daughter always struggled. I just couldn't understand why fat stuck to her while my other two children easily maintained their healthy weights.

As any mom understands, her frustration was my frustration. Her suffering was my suffering. Her joy was my joy. They still are. Oftentimes, we mothers feel more, learn more, and grow more through our own children than we do through our own experiences. In fact, their experiences are indeed our experiences.

Nika is one of my three greatest teachers, one of my three greatest growth experiences, and one of my three greatest joys and loves. Because of her I keenly sense how you feel about your body, hopelessly trapped in too many layers.

I don't claim to know you. We are all different. But as different as we are, we all have one thing in common – we deserve to feel good about ourselves. Being held hostage by fat for far too long doesn't make us feel good about ourselves.

Unbeknownst to me at the time, that moment with my 8-year-old daughter and her pain-provoking pink pants was pivotal in my life. A seed was planted. And that seed, fertilized by life's experiences, sprouted into that specific focus of my passion and my life's purpose: You – and helping you get into your pants.

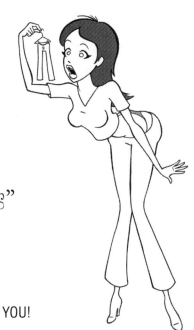

Chapter 1

Turning "Those Pants" into "Your Pants"

- It's all about YOU!

- What to expect as you're shifting from the inside out

- Why this plan will work for you

- A sneak peek at 10+10 For Life®

IT'S ALL ABOUT YOU!

We all have that pair of pants somewhere in our memory or still buried in our closet. Those pants we wore on a first date twenty-five years ago, or those that we haven't worn since before we had kids. Those pants that we saved for years, and every New Year's we resolve to fit into again before summer. But it just never happens. Finally, we realize we'll never be able to wear those pants again and donate them to Goodwill. After three decades as a health care practitioner helping individuals achieve a higher level of health, I've realized that the desire to get into those very pants cries out louder to us than any doctor, talk show host, latest diet book, nagging mother or spouse, or fear of looming diseases.

That's the purpose of this book: to help you turn "those pants" back into "your pants."

So let's start with the hard truth: it's tough to lose weight – sometimes impossibly tough. Moreover, it's even tougher to keep weight off once it's gone. All too often weight loss is a process that leaves you feeling like a hopeless failure. Again and again and again. Year after year after year. Nothing seems to work for good.

One thing's for sure – you're sick of it: sick of the weight, sick of thinking about food, sick of stressing about every morsel that goes into your mouth, and sick of feeling crummy about yourself with no end in sight. After the many times you've endured the scale's telltale ups, downs, and, ultimately, ups, you've made the conscious choice to step into the weight-woe arena once more. That takes guts.

I can assure you this time is different. You're no longer interested in a short, 3-month or 6-month sprint of counting, measuring, fussing, starving, and depriving. That works, until it doesn't. How well you know. Weight may leave for a while, but when you start eating "normally," it returns – with a vengeance.

This time, you're in it for the long haul – the long haul of your life. And you want it all – not just to lose weight, but to build up your energy, your health, and your "self." You crave that seeing-is-believing reward for your efforts: the simple pleasure of getting into your pants.

I, and all of your fans, applaud you. Your courage and bull-dog determination are inspiring. Those pants are going to be yours – one mindful step at a time.

WHAT TO EXPECT AS YOU'RE SHIFTING FROM THE INSIDE OUT

This program, 10+10 for Life®, is not about trapping you into the kind of rigid food box that you can't wait to get out of before you even begin. It's not all or nothing. It's not about success or failure. It's not about guilt.

It's about shifting – shifting your thinking about food, your choices, your habits, and, gradually, gently shifting your everyday life. After a while, the effort-full magically transforms into the effort-less. And then you're free from the layers, inside and out. Can you imagine what that feeling would be like – to be trim, fit, energetic, loving life, fully present, and grateful to be all that you are?

10+10 for Life® is simple common sense. It teaches you how to get the most nutrition for your calorie buck. That doesn't mean it's always easy. Change is never easy, especially when it comes to food. However, it's doable with reasonable goals, in reasonable time, and with wiggle room. (We all need wiggle room.)

10+10 can open up new doors of awareness, one after the other:

- You can consistently lose weight, eating as much as you want of the best-for-you foods.

- You can get full and completely satisfied, without feeling constantly hungry or deprived.

- You can consciously make better food choices, and even like those choices.

- You can control cravings instead of cravings controlling you.

- You can "cheat" guilt-free – the only slip up is to give up.

- You can boost your energy and lift your attitude.

- You can prepare one simple meal for you and your family, without too many grumbles from the sidelines.

- You can make grocery shopping simple, fun, and list-free.

- You can "get up off of that thing" and even enjoy it.

- You can tune out the nay-sayers and tune into your own voice and what works best for you.

- You can claim self-responsibility for your weight, body, and life, fueling self-empowerment.

- You can feel good about you!

WHY THIS PLAN WILL WORK FOR YOU

Bottom line: This plan will work for you because it's practical, flexible, and personalized to fit you. It's based on years of practice, research, and proven results. It will provide a smooth transition from where you *are now* to where you *want to go*. Most importantly, it's the best thing you can do for your body – both inside and out.

And, although the program results in lasting weight loss, the logic behind 10+10 for Life® centers on your health needs. Specifically, it focuses on the fact that, in spite of all the confusion out there about good foods, bad foods, and fat, there is no confusion about the answer to this simple question:

"Which foods prevent cancer?"

Come on, we all know this one: whole, fresh fruits and vegetables, of course! And, not surprisingly, these are the very same foods that fight heart disease, stroke, diabetes, arthritis, fatigue, depression, digestive problems – and too much fat. Fruits and vegetables are our disease and weight warriors and our energy and health heroes. And, not surprisingly, these are the very same foods on which 10+10 for Life® is based.

If we all know these foods are the best for us, why aren't we already building our meals on fruits and vegetables? Simple. We weren't taught to. We were raised with the "one apple a day and a side dish of canned peas" mentality.

I've never read or heard anyone say that beef, chicken, cheese, milk, eggs, brown-colored white bread, pasta, and dried-up cereals from cardboard boxes prevented cancer. Have you? Yet, we were deeply conditioned to love those foods. We center our meals, our days, and, indeed, our lives on them. Is it any wonder so many of us are sick, tired, fat, and frustrated?

How about making the very first shift right now? Are you game?

The first and most important shift in 10+10 for Life® is to learn how to center your meals on the best-for-you-foods first and then fill in the blanks with the other foods. I'll explain more about this concept in chapter 5, but I feel it's important for you to know up front that this lifestyle change is not about sacrificing. It's not a test of wills. There are no pie-in-the-sky proclamations of giving up your food faves forever and ever and ever. That's not going to happen anyway so why go there?

This is just a simple shift in food priorities. Curious? Let's get specific.

A SNEAK PEAK AT 10+10 FOR LIFE®

First, we'll take a look at the scary truth about how you got to where you are now and why this program is different from the diets that have failed you in the past. Then, I'll lead you through a fun and eye-opening self-assessment of your present level of health. Using this assessment tool, I'll help you create personalized weight and health goals for yourself. With your new goals in mind, you will learn about the 10+10 program in depth. I'll answer a lot of your questions and help you side-step predictable roadblocks while you tailor this plan to your life. Lastly, I'll help you plan your first week of the program, and give you some tips about how to stay on track. After all, this is all about you!

As for your specific food choices…well, once you have the will and the direction, the way is much easier. Since fruits and vegetables provide the best nutrition for your calorie buck, they will make up the bulk of your food choices. So, let's discuss them first. It's important to know how you can add more of these foods to your breakfast, lunch, dinner, and snacks.

Here's a super-short snapshot of your 10+10 food day. The details about what to eat and the reasoning behind the food choices will be discussed in later chapters.

Breakfast

Eat your choice of whole, fresh fruits, staggered throughout the morning, to keep you full and satisfied. And, yes, fruit can fill you up – if you eat enough! To give you an idea, I eat as many as 10 whole fruits from the time I wake up until noonish – as in two apples, three oranges, three bananas, a bunch of grapes (no, I don't count them), and a whole cantaloupe. No, I'm not kidding. I really eat that much. And, if you want eggs, toast, pancakes, or whatever your breakfast favorites happen to be, by all means, go ahead. Just be sensible – once a week, not once a day.

Lunch

Fill up on a 10-veggie, green-leafy salad with an oil-free dressing. For variety, you could try a power-packed vegetable sandwich with an avocado or hummus (garbanzo bean) spread, a veggie wrap, or homemade veggie and bean soup. Does this mean you can never, ever eat one of your traditional sandwich favorites with meat, cheese, and mayo on brown-colored white bread? Not at all. Remember, you have wiggle room.

When you want snacks between meals, grab some raw, unsalted nuts and seeds, or cut up vegetables or fresh fruit.

Dinner

Fill up in this order: First, start with the best-for-you foods – a medium-size veggie salad. Second, eat lightly steamed vegetables, such as broccoli, cauliflower, and asparagus. Third, add to your meal cooked, more filling vegetables, like potatoes, yams, or winter squash or a whole grain, like brown rice and/or beans. Fourth, and very last, *if* you still feel hungry, add traditional dinner dishes, like beef, chicken, turkey, pork, lamb, fish, or pasta.

THE POINT OF IT ALL

The whole idea is to fill *up* throughout the day on the best-for-you foods first, then fill *in* with the worst-for-you foods last. That way, your hunger drive will be satisfied and your stomach filled with more nutrients and fewer calories, leaving less room and desire for high-fat, high-cholesterol, low-nutrient, low-fiber, and/or high-calorie old-time favorites.

By the end of each day, you'll be amazed how many fruits and vegetables you've eaten, usually close to 10 whole fruits and more than 10 different vegetables. Now, that's what I call food power.

Thus the name: 10+10 for Life® – that's 10 fruits and 10 vegetables each day for life!

HOW TOUGH IS TOUGH?

Now that the 10+10 principles have been introduced, let's tackle your self doubt head-on.

Is it tough to shed pounds and keep them off over the long haul? You bet. But tough as it is, it can be easier than you've experienced in the past, *if* you're ready.

10+10 for Life® offers a simple, sensible plan with doable direction and, most importantly, hope – hope that you can step into your body-dream-come-true and stay there.

All you have to do now is make the commitment to yourself to give 10+10 a go. Give it a fair chance, let's say for one month. Then, see how you feel about the program and yourself.

You've got nothing to lose – but weight – and everything to gain – like getting into those pants!

WHAT YOU NOW KNOW...

You can get into your pants while building health if you:

- Shift your thinking, food choices, and lifestyle habits.

- Eat the best-for-you foods first – fresh fruits and vegetables.

- Believe those pants can be your pants by transitioning to 10+10 for Life® – a nutritious, simple, flexible plan tailored just for you.

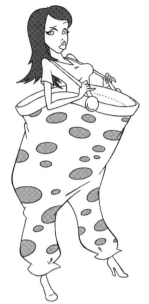

Chapter 2

Stuck in Big-Girl Pants

- We haven't had a chance since birth, and we're still stuck

- Fat – the real deal on the silent enemy that kills

NO CHANCE SINCE BIRTH AND STILL STUCK

You're stuck in big-girl pants, and as hard as you've tried, you're unable to get rid of them for good. You can't even figure out how you allowed yourself to get stuck in those darn pants in the first place. You hate them.

Stop beating yourself up! I'm here to tell you that you may not be the only one to blame for your struggle with weight. And no, I'm not talking about nature vs. nurture. Regardless of your genes, the truth is you haven't had a fighting chance since birth. Not that you're entirely off the hook, you're a big girl now and ultimately the one responsible for you. But give yourself a break. The deck was stacked against you – big time! After all, you were birthed from the loins of our culture, and our culture created monsters – food monsters. And, just like all of us food monsters, you want to eat what you want, when you want it, without regard to big, fat consequences.

The result: You and a whole nation – indeed, an entire world – of people who are overweight, out of shape, tired, plagued by aches and pains, ripe for diseases, and the worst part of all, terribly unhappy with themselves.

Let's start at the very beginning, so you can see for yourself how you got where you are and why you should shift at least a little of the blame off yourself.

Baby Bottle Blues and Little Jar Gooze

If you're a baby boomer, chances are you weren't fed nature's perfect food for baby humans – mama's milk. If you were, lucky you. I wasn't that fortunate, nor were my five brothers and sisters. More than likely you, too, were given a warmed-up bottle filled with the accepted, man-made formula of the day.

As you got a bit older, the formula was replaced by cow's milk – the perfect food for baby cows that can gain up to 600 pounds the first year, but not the perfect food for baby people. Only people milk is perfect for baby people.

To complement the bottle were your mother's best friends – little jarred baby foods filled with cooked, strained meats, cereals, vegetables, and fruits, often with added salt, sugar, and chemicals.

So, nature's perfect food for Baby You was replaced first by artifi-cially-made concoctions of fake milk and then by moo-juice and over-processed adult-food goo.

There you were – just a baby – and already filling up on foods that stopped your hunger pains, but were inferior in nutrition. That's not a great way to start a healthy, lifelong relationship with food.

Welcome to America, Baby You, and your future challenges with food, weight, health, and your "self."

Weaned on the Not-So-Fab Four

When you were old enough to jump from the baby bottle and baby jars to big-people food, you were given the same foods that all big people in our culture ate – foods from the good, ole', not-so-fab Four Food Groups, fully embraced by doctors, teachers, government officials, and the most powerfully influential person of all, your mother.

Oh, yes, we're all very familiar with the Four Food Groups: (1) meats/fish, (2) milk/dairy products, (3) grains/breads/cereals, and (4) fruits/vegetables. The food pyramid, which still spotlights meat, fish, dairy, grains, breads, and cereals, has since replaced the Four Food Groups. Sure, both the new and the old guidelines include fresh fruit and vegetables, but let's be honest – they were, and still are, forgotten underlings. You never ate enough fresh fruits and vegetables growing up, and you probably still don't. Neither do your kids and grandkids.

Take breakfast for instance. You were weaned on dried-up cereal or instant oatmeal with sugar and milk, as well as eggs, bacon, and white toast with butter and jam. Pancakes or waffles, smothered in butter and Aunt Jemima's sweetness, were a likely weekend treat.

Your lunchbox featured peanut butter and jelly on Wonder Bread or bologna with cheese, mayo, and perhaps a piece of lettuce. Rounding out your midday meal was every kid's favorite vegetable: the potato chip. Or maybe a pickle, an apple, or cookies. A sugary juice drink from your thermos chased it all down. Or you bought a carton of milk (better yet – chocolate milk) with the few, precious pennies your mom pressed into your hand as you ran out the door. If you were lucky enough to buy lunch at school, it was probably hot and mushy and came with one of those little ice cream treats eaten with a flat wooden spoon. After school, you rushed home to snack time – graham crackers and milk.

At the dinner table, meat claimed superstar status. Think back a minute. What was your mother's response to your predictable, pesky question, "What's for dinner, Mom?" Do chicken, hamburgers, beef stew, pot roast, meat loaf, pork chops, or chuck steak sound familiar? Cooked-to-death vegetables, like canned corn or frozen lima beans (yuck!) relegated to lowly side dishes were never mentioned. After all, they probably tasted horrible, so why mention them? Along with your meat-dominated dinner, you drank milk or sweet lemonade made from frozen concentrate. *If* you cleaned your plate like a good girl (and you were well-behaved besides), dessert was your rightful reward – maybe even two big scoops of Neapolitan ice cream or freshly baked, home-made chocolate chip cookies.

So I ask you, where in your day were the weight warriors and health heroes hiding – fresh fruits and vegetables?

The answer: they were snubbed out by the more popular celebrities of the Not-So-Fab Four – meat, seafood, cheese, milk, eggs, breads, and dried-up cereals.

If fresh fruits and vegetables were included in your day, their presence was miniscule. Can you imagine asking your mom, "What's for dinner?" and her responding with, "A vegetable salad, yams, roasted peppers, broccoli, black beans, and a side of chicken"?

The fact was, a small serving of frozen peas, canned, sugary, peaches, a slice of tomato on a meat sandwich, or maybe a fresh apple were enough fruits and vegetables to keep a growing child toddling around and your mother feeling good about what she was feeding her family. However, skimping on fruits and vegetables didn't help keep the pounds off later or ward off diseases that crept up and destroyed our bodies and lives.

"Mmmm Good, Mmmm Good..."

And, as if the home-cooked meals weren't bad enough, along came so-called modern, convenience foods – refined, processed, packaged, preserved, artificial, and instant foods that fit nicely into the parameters of the Four Food Groups. Your mom never thought to question how good they were for you. All she knew was that everyone ate them, and they made her life a whole lot easier.

Campbell's chicken noodle soup, toasted Velveeta cheese sandwiches, Kraft macaroni and cheese, lickable Oreo cookies, and Betty Crocker's devil's food chocolate cake became household favorites (and probably can still conjure up those warm fuzzy feelings).

Fast + Cheap + Big + Good = Big FAT Trouble

Then, after the barrage of bad foods at home, that final, knock-down blow in the weight arena came from fast foods – the ultimate in convenience for the hectic lifestyle of the working mom. These super fast, super cheap, super big, and super yummy foods snuck into your life and added another huge dimension to your already growing proportions and compromised body.

Now you were in a real fix – adding quickie burgers, fries, shakes, pop, pizza, and fried chicken to the already high-fat, high-cholesterol, high-sugar, high-salt American foods that had been a part of your life since your first memory.

And the bad news of fast foods got worse. The average fast food meal back in the '60s was about 590 calories. Today the super-sized burger, fries, and soda can reach over 2000 calories! Whew – that's more calories than most women require in a whole day, not just one meal! No wonder we're in big trouble.

Adding layers to the layers, sweets, salty snacks, junk foods, and drinks in all shapes and sizes became more and more accessible and popular, thanks to advertising and marketing aimed at silencing the whines of hungry children and selling convenience to the working mom.

Like a Good Little Girl, You Did As You Were Told

Are you starting to get the big picture now? With all the competition from fast, easy, tasty, and "cool" foods, fresh fruits and vegetables didn't stand a chance. Nor did you. And how many hundreds, maybe thousands, of times have you beaten yourself up with nagging, negative self-talk, like: "I knew better than to eat that. But I ate it anyway. What's wrong with me? I must be weak or lazy or undisciplined or just plain dumb or all of the above to let my weight get so out of hand."

Quit the self-abuse and guilt! We all make bad choices. You are no more weak, lazy, undisciplined, or dumb than the rest of us mere mortals. You are simply the product of a lifetime of conditioning, eating what your mother and an entire culture told you to eat. You grew up believing that your mother's way of feeding you was the best way of eating. Period. No questions asked.

It's difficult to break free from those chains. But certainly not impossible. No, you haven't had a chance since birth. But the good news? You do now.

FAT — THE REAL DEAL ON THE SILENT ENEMY THAT KILLS

For as isolating and ostracizing as fat can be, you are not alone in your misery. You have lots of company. We are facing a crisis – a huge fat crisis. And it isn't just America getting too big for her britches. Fat has gone global.

Here are a few frightening international facts about fat:

- There are now more overweight people on the planet (1 billion) than starving people (600 million).

- Today, over 300 million people are obese (thirty pounds or more overweight). In 1995, 200 million were obese. We're growing – and fast.

- Obesity has tripled in Europe in the last twenty years.

- Obesity doesn't just affect modern, industrialized nations – over 115 million people are obese in developing nations. Today, in most African countries, more women are overweight than underweight.

- In China, one in five adults is now overweight. That's 264 million people in China alone!

And what about us here in America? As smart, savvy, rich, and sophisticated as we are, we seem clueless when it comes to our growing girth. Here's proof:

- Americans are the fattest people on the planet, with approximately 66% of our population overweight, and 34% obese.

- U.S. health care costs are 36% higher for obese people than for people who maintain a healthy weight.

- According to the National Institute of Health, obesity costs in lives and dollars: a twofold increase in mortality and over 100 billion dollars a year.

Fat Does More Than Look Bad

You may be unhappy with the size of your pants, but the bad news gets worse – your pants may be bigger than you think. When you step into a size 12 pants today, those same pants would have been a size 14 or larger twenty-five or thirty years ago. Yes, the clothing industry actually changed their size standards to accommodate our growing bodies. That means that there's an even bigger increase in the average women's size than statistics show.

Worse than the ever-widening of our pants is the enormous increase in disability, chronic diseases, and early death associated with carrying around too much fat. These debilitating and deadly diseases include type 2 diabetes, heart disease, high blood pressure, high cholesterol, stroke, gall bladder diseases, certain cancers (uterine, ovarian, breast, cervical, prostate, colorectal, pancreatic, liver, kidney), osteoarthritis, and degenerative joint disease, leading to knee and hip replacements.

I remind you. Disability and diseases don't just happen to other people – they can happen to you too! And, as your weight goes up, so do your chances for getting sick, and worse. As Dr. John McDougall says, the fat you eat is the fat you wear. That same fat maims and kills. See for yourself and be alarmed:

- 400,000 deaths every year in America can be directly attributed to too much weight.

- Obese adults significantly increase their risk for type 2 diabetes, hypertension, heart disease, cancer, high triglycerides, high cholesterol, sleep apnea, gallstones, lung disease, gastrointestinal diseases, and degenerative arthritis.

- 20 pounds of extra fat at twenty years old to middle age doubles the risk of postmenopausal breast cancer.

- The risk for colon cancer increases by three to four times in obese people.

- Compared to eating no poultry, eating poultry once a week increases risk of colon cancer by 55%. Eating poultry four times a week increases colon cancer by 200-300%.

- Too much weight has surpassed smoking as the nation's leading cause of preventable death.

- 80% of people with type 2 diabetes are overweight.

- Women with a BMI of 30 (approximately thirty pounds overweight) increase their relative risk of developing type 2 diabetes by 3000 percent – a greater correlation than the 2000 percent correlation between smoking and lung cancer. Read these stats once again. It's shocking!

- Diabetes increases the risk of stroke and fatal heart attacks by two to four times and is the leading cause of blindness in adults and end-stage kidney disease. Sixty percent of all lower limb amputations result from diabetes.

- Risk of heart disease is two to three times higher in obese people.

- Obesity among vegetarians is 6% and among vegans, who consume no animal products, 2%.

WHAT ABOUT OUR FUTURE — OUR PRECIOUS CHILDREN?

The most heart-wrenching facts of all concern our children. It's one thing to destroy our own bodies. It's quite another to destroy our children's:

- According to the U.S. Surgeon General, overweight children doubled from 1982 to 2002 and tripled for adolescents.

- 25% of American children are overweight, as reported in the International Journal of Epidemiology, October 2005.

- According to the Centers for Disease Control, 50% of American children will be overweight by 2010, and 30 to 40% of those who are children today will get diabetes in their lifetimes.

- One soft drink or sweetened drink a day increases a child's risk of becoming obese by 60%. That doesn't even count all the other high fat, high sugar, high calorie foods and pseudo-foods that children put into their bodies every day.

- Almost one-third of American children eat fast food every day.

THE Simple Solution

The scariest part of these stats is that our fat problem is mushrooming out of control. And the experts know it. In their efforts to short stop the worldwide overweight epidemic and its inevitable consequences, the World Health Organization, along with the American Cancer Society, the American Heart Association, the U.S. government, research scientists, and some of our own doctors, now recommend this simple food guide:

Eat more fruits and vegetables, fewer animal products, and less fat and sugar!

Whoa! What a concept. Eat real, whole foods – fresh fruits and vegetables – that provide all the nutrients necessary for human health and vitality, as well as keep our weight where it should be. With all due respect, I can't help but wonder how many hundreds of experts, collective years of education, high-powered meetings, and billions of dollars it took to come up with that conclusion.

Somehow, plain ole' common sense got lost along the way – and all of us right along with it! And unfortunately, when it comes to food and weight, we are still lost.

And the real tragedy? As common sense as it is, the simple fruit and vegetable solution continues to be ignored, no matter who champions it.

Whether or not you're listening to these expert voices of the day, one thing is certain. They DO NOT promote "fad diets" as the solution for our health and weight woes, and for good reason. Diets… don't…work! In the next chapter, I'll explain why.

WHAT YOU NOW KNOW...

- Since birth we were taught to fill up on the wrong foods.

- Americans are clueless – we're the fattest people on the planet, killing ourselves with our own choices.

- The Simple Solution for getting into your pants: eat more fruits and vegetables, fewer animal products, and less fat, salt, and sugar.

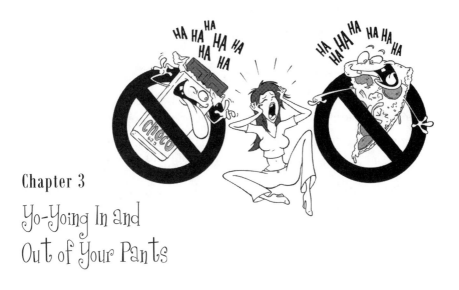

Chapter 3

Yo-Yoing In and Out of Your Pants

- You didn't fail; the diets failed you
- What's the difference between 10+10 and a diet?

YOU DIDN'T FAIL; THE DIETS FAILED YOU

Okay. Fess up. There's no denying – you don't eat right or exercise nearly enough. And the proof is right in front, and below, your nose – the fat that you hate hanging onto your hips, thighs, butt, tummy, and arms. And, if you're like most of my clients, you've been intimate with almost every diet known to mankind and disappointed with the results every time.

Sure, sometimes you didn't try that hard or gave up way too soon, but even when you were geared up and gave it your all, the ride on the diet-go-round dittoed every dizzying diet ride before and ended in the same frustrating fat place it started.

Round and Round on the Diet-go-Round

If I were a bettin' gal, I'd put money on the fact that all of your diet routines went something like this: You planned. You measured. You counted. You sacrificed. You starved. You craved. You snuck (silly girl, as if you can really sneak from yourself). You cheated. You denied. You guilted. You beat yourself up (you're a master at that). You lost. You gained. You lost. You gained. You plateaued. You plateaued. You plateaued and, f-i-n-a-l-l-y, you lost – a pound. Then you went to a friend's house for dinner and gained two pounds back.

Then you kept gaining, pound by pound, until you were right back where you started, or even heavier. Your mood yo-yoed right along with the number on the scale. The scale went down, your mood went up. The scale went up, your mood went down. That little number glaring at you every morning and whether you could wiggle yourself into those pants dictated how you felt about yourself. Then, eventually, you came to the realization that you are an adult. You are the way you are. And, you're going to eat what you want from now on because the agony of it all isn't worth it. You aren't seeing results, and you're miserable.

Even before you started the diet, and then throughout, you mourned what you "had to" give up. Then when you started, you couldn't wait to eat those restricted foods. You felt deprived, even sorry for yourself. And then the predictable happened, just as it always did before. You quit! After all, you're human. You can put up with self-imposed hunger, restriction, and entrapment for only so long before you bolt.

After you realized the diet didn't work (just like all the rest of them), you vowed to ban diets forever. That worked until that next quick-fix, fat-melting, no-fail diet came along, appealing to your sense of desperation to be slim and luring you into believing that it would somehow be different from the dozens of diets you had tried before. Then you climbed back aboard the diet-go-round, going round and round, with the scale going up and down, and ultimately up. And you ended, yet again, feeling badly about yourself.

Now how does a capable, strong woman like you become such a failure when it comes to something as simple as eating? The good news: you didn't fail; the diets failed you. Let's figure out why, so you can hop off the diet-go-round and get into those pants – for good.

The Fat Business Fails Its Way to Fat Success

In the United States, we spend billions of dollars every year on the business of losing weight; yet look at how many of us continue to battle the bulge. It doesn't take a genius to see that those quick, easy fixes, called diets, may work – for a short time – but are utter failures over the long haul of life. If diets worked, America would be sleek and svelte. But, as we can all see, America is anything but slim.

Since diets have a ninety-five percent or more failure rate, meaning all weight lost is gained back within three years, you would think that the diet business would go fat-belly up. Can you imagine any other business staying afloat with such a dismal rate of success? There are dozens of big, new diets each year, but Americans keep getting fatter and fatter.

So why does the weight-loss business continue to flourish? Simple. It feeds on the desperation and gullibility of Americans, especially us women, dying to be thin and look like all those ultra-thin, ultra-gorgeous, ultra-sexy babes flashed everywhere from magazine covers to advertisements to television and movies.

We can't help but buy into the illusion and the hope that the next diet will work. Not only do we want it to work, but we want it to be fast and effortless. Like magic!

Come on, we all know better. Losing weight and maintaining your health is hard work. Just like raising a child or pursuing a career, it requires a lifelong commitment to learning, planning, growing, and good old-fashion elbow grease.

Anyone who tells you it's easy is trying to sell you a new diet.

But Why Don't Quick-fix Diets Work?

The driving force behind any raved diet-of-the-day is to get you to lose weight fast – not permanently. The quicker and more effortless, the more profitable because it feeds into our desperation to lose weight *now*. The promise of melting fat away while you sleep sells books and programs, thus lining pockets with cash. Sensible, slow, steady weight loss is a tough sell to a whole culture of people who want what they want when they want it – if not sooner.

Whether a diet preaches high protein, low fat, low carb, high carb, prepackaged diet meals, diet shakes three times a day, or baby-sized starvation portions, the real truth is that weight gain or loss is ultimately dictated by one very simple math equation:

(Calories IN) - (Calories OUT) = The FAT You Wear

Sure, any diet that drastically cuts calories can work for a while. But, in the end, all diets share one common flaw: they are not designed to work permanently. Therefore, as soon as you get fed up with the diet and do the inevitable, you abandon it. The weight boomerangs back with a vengeance. Sound familiar?

Even if you possess the super human will power needed to make a diet permanent, unless it centers on the best-for-you-foods, it's not good for your health. When you significantly slash calories or cut out a major nutrient (yes, like carbs!), you are depriving your body of necessary nutrients. That's akin to draining your car of gas without replenishing it. After a while, it stops running.

So the next logical question you may be asking is: "What distinguishes 10+10 for Life® from the diet-rave-of-the day?"

Let's compare the fundamental differences to give you a clear understanding of 10+10 for Life®. Then you can decide for yourself whether you and 10+10 are the right fit – just like you want those pants to be.

WHAT'S THE DIFFERENCE BETWEEN 10+10 AND A DIET?

I'll be perfectly honest. 10+10 for Life® is not a quick fix. If that's what you're looking for, then this is not the program for you. However, if you want to consistently and permanently lose weight the health-smart way – by fueling up on our weight warriors and health heroes – 10+10 offers a simple, effective solution for you. If you have the want and the will, it will show you the way.

If your burning desire is to lose weight while still building your health, you can accomplish that *if* you have the want and the will to follow 10+10 to the letter. It goes without saying, the more wiggle-room you take from the 10+10 guidelines, the longer it will take to lose the weight. And that's okay – your pace is your choice. You can still get there.

YOU DECIDE: 10+10 FOR LIFE® VERSUS THE TYPICAL DIET-OF-THE-DAY

1. **Diets** promote the myth that to lose weight you must control your hunger drive. When you can't, you feel inherently weak, lacking will power and self-control.

   10+10 teaches you that the hunger drive is natural and normal and cannot be controlled. It's an instinct. And, like all instincts – thirst, sleeping, breathing, sex – it keeps you alive and the human race thriving. To feel full and satisfied, you must satisfy your hunger drive, not wage war with it.

2. **Diets** trap you into a rigid diet box with built-in food laws. If you're a conforming, good girl, and you stay in the box and abide by the laws, you'll lose weight. If you're a rebellious, bad girl and break free from the box, you'll gain any lost weight right back, and often more.

   10+10 opens your awareness and helps you build a foundation of food facts that shift your thinking about what you eat and why you eat it, freeing you to make better daily food choices gradually and replace the old habits that fuel your weight woes with new habits that shed the layers, inside and out.

3. **Diets** encourage cheating, followed by guilt and bad feelings about yourself. After all, who can stay trapped in a diet box forever?

   10+10 builds "cheating" into its three simple rules. It's called "wiggle room," and it teaches you how to cheat and still lose weight.

4. **Diets** make you feel weak, undisciplined, lazy, or all of the above, if you slip up.

   10+10 says that the only slip up is to give up. So-called slipping up is totally normal and natural for all of us mere mortals. When you get off track, there's no need for self-floggings. You let it go – what's done is done – and get right back on track.

5. **Diets** make you bid a tearful, final farewell to your favorite food friends, making you feel deprived and lonely – until you can't stand it and sneak them back into your life.

   10+10 emphasizes the positive action steps of adding new best-for-you food friends to your day, not subtracting and sacrificing your old food pals. No matter how clear your intentions, chances are you're not going to give them up forever anyway, so why pretend otherwise and set yourself up for failure?

6. **Diets** restrict calories and portions, leaving you hungry, making you want more, and building that food frenzy to a height that consumes your thoughts and your life.

   10+10 gives you the freedom to eat until you're full and satisfied. When you're hungry again, you eat again – the best for you foods first.

7. **Diets** often limit one of the major nutrient groups – carbohydrates, proteins, or fats. This inevitably limits your body's ability to get the nutrients it needs, and leads to cravings and food binges when you just can't take the deprivation any more.

10+10 offers all the nutrients, without counting or fussing. It ensures you have appropriate amounts of carbohydrates, proteins, fats, vitamins, minerals, enzymes, fiber, and micronutrients necessary for human health.

8. **Diets** emphasize high fat and high cholesterol foods, and even added oils, which all add fat to your fat and clog up your arteries and veins, making you ripe for disabilities and diseases.

    10+10 emphasizes naturally low-fat, low-calorie foods that naturally eliminate extra body fat, while preventing diseases and boosting health.

9. **Diets** mess up your metabolism, which is critical for efficiently burning calories and regulating weight. If you've been a long-time dieter, perhaps you've noticed how hard it is to lose weight, even severely cutting calories. Yet, the weight flies back on the moment you stray from the diet. What's up with that?

    Calorie-restricted yo-yo diets, which promote rapid weight loss and weight gain, simulate starvation to your body. So, when you go into diet mode, your body thinks it's going to starve, and metabolism slows to conserve energy (you burn less and save more). The result: painfully slow weight loss, if any at all.

    On the flip side, when you pile on the calories again, your body says, "Yippee! She's not starving me anymore. I better stock up reserves (fat!) as quickly as I can just in case she starves me again." The very unfair result: seemingly blink-of-an-eye weight gain after all those painfully drawn-out weeks and months of slaving and starving to lose those pounds. Of course, it's more complicated than that when you get into the actual body physiology, but you get the idea. In fact, you've probably experienced it for yourself.

10+10 promotes natural weight loss that occurs by eating foods that are nutrient-dense and calorie-low to help you break through your body's self-preservation mode that hangs onto weight. Once you reach your ideal weight, staying the 10+10 course keeps calories at a natural minimum, freeing you from the worry of weight gain. Again.

10. **Diets** zap your energy, making you tired and sometimes feeling depressed. They restrict those very foods that supply you with your most efficient sources of energy.

    10+10 provides you with an abundance of your best energy foods.

11. **Diets** intensify cravings for refined, bad-guy foods, which are empty of nutrition and high in calories. Diets deprive you of the very foods that satisfy your hunger drive and control cravings.

    10+10 crushes cravings because it centers your food day on those very foods that fill you up, satisfying your hunger drive.

12. **Diets** consume time with the involved planning and meticulous measuring, counting, weighing, and fussing in strict compliance with the diet's laws.

    10+10 saves time, once you become well-acquainted with 10+10 and get into the 10+10 groove. It's a very simple plan, with only three easy-to-remember rules, minimal food preparation, and lots of variety to choose from.

13. **Diets** focus on satisfying immediate gratification and flash weight loss for that next class reunion. They do not steadily get you down to your ideal pant size and keep you there.

    10+10 teaches that with commitment, effort, simple direction, and hope, you can reach your ideal weight and maintain that weight for the rest of your life.

14. **Diets** completely ignore the primary purpose of food and basic nutrition – to build, maintain, and restore health for a long and purposeful life.

    10+10 wraps its entire program around the best foods for human health – the very foods that are also absolutely critical for losing weight and keeping it off forever.

    So there you have it – the 10+10 difference. The rest of this book will delve more deeply into the food-specifics of the program. But before we go there, it's important that you get a sense of where you're starting, in terms of weight and health, and where you *would like* to go. If you're ready to open yourself up to a new way of thinking, living, and looking in those pants, off we go to the Chapter 4 mirror for a bit of soul-searching.

WHAT YOU NOW KNOW...

- Diets don't work.

- 10+10 for Life® works because you:
    — fill up.
    — satisfy your hunger drive.
    — boost your energy.
    — add the best-for-you foods instead of subtracting, depriving, starving, and feeling guilty.
    — crush cravings with nutrient-rich, calorie-low foods.
    — save time – no more counting, measuring, weighing, and fussing.
    — get into your pants and feel good about yourself every step of the way.

Chapter 4

"Mirror, Mirror on the Wall, Make My Pants Fit After All"

- The Mirror Test – Your Moment of Truth
- The Healthy U Check-up

Just like any other journey, when charting your course to your ideal weight and health, your success depends on knowing your starting and ending points. In other words, where are you right now and where do you want to go?

In this chapter, you will learn practical, eye-opening (and maybe even fun) tools that will help you define your starting point and create your vision for yourself. The rest of the book will help you plot your course between those two points, however far apart or close together they may be.

THE MIRROR TEST — YOUR MOMENT OF TRUTH

After working with many women in my practice, I've realized that the true answers to questions about how we feel about our weight and ourselves can be hard to pin down.

The "Mirror Test" is a great springboard to start asking and answering the important questions we will discuss in this chapter. But I warn you, you have to be very bold to take this test. I know – I'm a middle-ager with lots of middle-age markers (no need for details), and the "Mirror Test" can be downright scary. Take a deep breath, relax, and don't even think about it – just go do it!

The Mirror Test

First, put on a pair of pants – the ones you wear a lot – and a top to go with them that hits you at your waist. (No, it can't go all the way down to your knees.) Then find a full-length mirror.

Stand in front of the mirror and do what most of us women do after we put on a pair of pants. Look at yourself face on, turn to one side, and check yourself out – your butt and stomach. Turn with your backside to the mirror and look over your shoulder. Well? What do you think? Are you happy with how you look? Sometimes, the hardest person to be honest with is oneself…Are you happy with how you look?

Okay, so much for the first part of the test. That was the easy part. Second, stand in front of that same full-length mirror, but this time…naked. That's right – clothes off!

What a good sport. Now look at yourself all the way around – front, side, and back views.

Do you love the reflection looking back at you? Yes? Do I see a smile? Or do I hear some noises – like a great big sigh and a few moans and groans? Wait a minute. Don't leave yet. Hang in there a bit longer.

Now look straight into your own eyes and ask yourself the question: "What are you sick and tired of? Be honest with yourself. It's just you – no one else is around. Are you tired of?

- Looking the way you do?

- Wearing **that** size pants?

- Feeling sluggish, worn out, and old – before your time?

- Getting winded after walking a half hour or less?

- Feeling left out because you can't play with your grandkids like you want to?

- Dealing with the rolls that get in your way – making it difficult to bend over and tie your shoes?

- Taking too many pills with no end in sight – a pill for blood pressure, another for cholesterol, two for diabetes, one for arthritis, more for depression, something for anxiety, something else for sleep, tablets for hot flashes, and a handful for pain?

- Being afraid of getting the same disease that snuck up on your mother or sister – like breast cancer or diabetes?

- Jiggling when you move, whether it is the flab in your thighs, bottom, or arms?

- Avoiding intimacy with your life partner because you're embarrassed and just don't feel sexy anymore?

- Thinking about food day in and day out?

- Feeling depressed?

- Feeling fat?

If you are fed up with any or all of these things, know that you aren't alone, and there is help. But first, ask yourself the most important question of all:

Do you *really* want to change?

WAIT! Don't answer yet. There's a lot more to this question than meets the eye.

Before you set your goals and start this journey – make sure you are setting yourself up for success. Here's a yes-or-no checklist to review before you give me your final answer.

1. Are you **really** committed to **you** and ready to **shift** your thinking, eating, exercise, and lifestyle gradually so you become the hero of your body-dream-come-true?

☐ Yes   ☐ No

2. Are you willing to learn about and then eat the best-for-you foods **first** each day? These are absolutely critical for you to reach your ideal weight and level of health and fitness.

☐ Yes   ☐ No

3. Are you willing to eat the not-so-good-for-you foods **last,** after the best-for-you foods, so you will automatically eat less of them without struggling?

☐ Yes   ☐ No

4. If you are not exercising for an hour every day, are you willing to increase your daily exercise?

☐ Yes ☐ No

5. Are you ready to stop making excuses as to why you can't take control of your weight and health?

☐ Yes ☐ No

Now…back to that question. <u>Do you **really** want to change?</u>

☐ Yes ☐ No

If so, congratulations! I'm here to help you. And, if not, don't set yourself up for failure – put this book in a safe place and pick it up later, when you're really ready to make that commitment to yourself.

So, for those of you willing and ready, let's move on to the <u>Healthy U Check-up</u> to get a better idea about who you are and what you want out of this program.

THE HEALTHY U CHECK-UP

The idea of the Healthy U Check-up is to get your starting point, set your goals, and then track your progress over the first several months of the 10+10 for Life® Program.

I'll warn you ahead of time that this self-assessment may take up to an hour to complete. So, if you don't have time right now, look at your calendar and make a date with yourself. Go ahead, I'll wait. Find your calendar. Now, promise yourself you'll follow through with your commitment. When you're ready, you can begin with the first section.

Part 1: Soul Searching

The "Mirror Test" got you thinking about how you feel about yourself and whether or not you're ready to make some shifts in your life to make you feel better. Let's dig a little deeper now. Take out a sheet of paper and a pen. Write today's date at the top. Now, think carefully about each question below and write down your honest answer. Don't just think about it. Actually write it down. It goes without saying, the more effort you put into completing the Healthy U Check-up, the more you will benefit.

1. What frustrates you about your weight, body, health, and/or fitness right now?

2. If you could snap your fingers and make **realistic,** instant changes in your weight, body, health, and/or fitness right now, what would you change? (No, brown eyes can't be blue!)

3. If you could snap your fingers and make **realistic** changes in your eating and exercise habits right now, what would you change (if anything)?

4. Dream of yourself **<u>five years</u>** from now.

    a. How many pounds would you like to weigh? (A key to weight loss and health gain is to keep your goal realistic. I recommend the doable weight-loss goal of 30 pounds, or less, in a year. That means 2.5 pounds or less per month.)____pounds

    b. How do you want to look? Use your own words, example: trim, fit, firm, muscular, younger, relaxed, sexy.

    c. How do you want to feel? Use your own words, example: light on my feet, full of energy, joyful from the inside out, pain-free, centered, in love with life, peaceful.

    d. List specific activities you can't participate in now because of weight or health issues that you would like to take up in the future (e.g. biking, walking a mile, playing with your grand-kids, cleaning the house without getting out of breath, volunteering, traveling, wearing a bathing suit, etc.)?

5. Dream of yourself **one year** from now.

a. How many pounds would you like to weigh **realistically**? (Again, realistic is key here. Remember, to be healthy and successful, I recommend that you aim for 2.5 pounds a month or less. That means 30 pounds in a year, at most.) ___ pounds

b. How do you want to look? Use your own specific words, example: trim, fit, firm, muscular, younger, relaxed, sexy.

c. How do you want to feel? Use your own specific words, example: light on my feet, full of energy, joyful from the inside out, pain-free, centered, in love with life, peaceful.

d. What **realistic** exercise program would you like to be enjoying? (Again, be realistic here, especially if exercise is not your favorite thing to do.) List each type of exercise, how many times a week, and how long for each session. If you're just starting out, choose an easier routine that you'll enjoy the most, as in walking. If you already exercise regularly, you may, or may not, want to upgrade your program and incorporate cardiovascular exercise, stretching, and strength training.

Example: walking 3-4 days a week for 40 minutes, two 1-hour sessions of yoga per week, and two 30-minute weight-lifting workouts with a personal trainer.

e. List specific activities you can't do now because of weight or health issues that you would like to be able to do within the following year. Be realistic here. Your goals for one year won't be as lofty as your five-year goals are.

6. At this point in your life, what diet, exercise, and lifestyle habits are you **unwilling** to change now, or ever, to make your body-dream-come-true? Be honest.

7. Now, look through your answers for Question 5. Will the habits you are unwilling to change restrict you from reaching your goals? (In other words, if you're unwilling to make any changes in your eating or exercise habits, then you will not reach your weight goals.)

☐ Yes   ☐ No

8. Do you honestly believe that you will be successful in meeting your goals?

☐ Yes   ☐ No

9. What is the most important thing you learned about yourself by answering these questions?

Part 2: Food and Beverage Audit

This part of the check-up will give you an idea of your starting point. As the months fly by, we'll take another look at these questions, and you'll see the progress you've made. Again, think carefully, and be honest with your answers. I suggest that you write directly in the book for Part 2, or make a photocopy and keep it in a safe place. This way, you won't have to copy the entire chart on separate paper.

Approximately how many servings of the following foods do you eat **per week?**

FOOD/BEVERAGE	TODAY'S DATE:	1 MONTH DATE:	3 MONTH DATE:	6 MONTH DATE:
Breakfast				
Oats (whole)				
*Whole grain bread/sprouted-grain bread				
**Fresh fruit				
Oats (instant)				
Cold cereal				
Refined-grain toast				
Bagels				
Pastries/muffins				
Pancakes/waffles				
Eggs				
Bacon, sausage, or other meat				
Yogurt				
Butter/margarine				
Jam/jelly				

Eating out or getting fast food				
**Water				
**Caffeine-free tea				
Milk (soy/rice)				
**Homemade veggie or fresh fruit juice/smoothie (no dairy)				
Store-bought juice				
Coffee or caffeinated tea				
Cow's milk				
Protein drinks				
Lunch				
Veggie sandwich, no cheese				
*Whole grain/sprouted-grain bread/tortilla/pocket bread				
Homemade veggie or bean soup				
**Vegetable salad				
**Raw vegetables (not in salad)				
Cooked, fresh vegetables				
Cooked, frozen vegetables				
**Fresh fruit				
**Raw, unsalted nuts and seeds				
Dried fruit (used sparingly)				
Sandwich with meat				
Veggie + cheese sandwich				
Refined-grain bread/tortillas				
Cooked, canned vegetables				
Pasta				
Soup with meat or dairy				

Canned fruit				
Dessert				
Eating out or getting fast food				
**Water				
**Caffeine-free tea				
Milk (soy/rice)				
**Homemade veggie or fresh fruit juice/smoothie (no dairy)				
Store-bought juice				
Coffee or caffeinated tea				
Cow's milk				
Protein drinks				
Soft drinks (soda/pop)				
Dinner				
*Whole grain/sprouted-grain bread/tortillas				
Tofu or meat substitute				
**Brown rice				
**Veggie or bean soup				
**Vegetable salad				
**Fresh, raw veggies (not in salad)				
**Cooked, fresh vegetables				
Cooked, frozen veggies				
**Potatoes/yams/winter squash				
**Fresh fruit				
Dried fruit (used sparingly)				
Meat (beef, poultry, pork, lamb)				
Seafood				

Soup with meat or dairy				
Cheese				
Refined-grain bread/tortillas				
Pasta				
White rice				
Cooked, canned veggies				
Canned fruit				
Dessert				
Eating out or getting fast food				
**Water				
**Caffeine-free tea				
Milk (soy/rice)				
**Homemade veggie or fresh fruit juice/smoothie (no dairy)				
Store-bought juice				
Coffee or caffeinated tea				
Cow's milk				
Protein drinks				
Soft drinks (soda/pop)				
Alcohol				
Snacks/Miscellaneous				
**Raw, unsalted nuts				
**Fruits/vegetables				
**Homemade fruit/veggie juice/ smoothie (no dairy)				
Chips				
Candy				
Salty snacks				

Salted nuts or seeds				
Refined-grain bread/tortillas				
Sweets/pastries				
Chocolate				
Crackers				
Sports drinks/soft drinks				

Whole Grain Bread - Remember, brown bread does not mean whole grain! (Often, this bread is merely white bread with caramel coloring to make it look healthier.) Always read the ingredients. For our purposes, a bread is considered whole grain if it satisfies one or both of the following requirements: (1) Whole wheat flour (not just wheat flour) is the only flour ingredient listed, (2) A whole grain is listed as the first ingredient, and the bread has a minimum of 2 grams of fiber per serving.

** *The double asterisk indicates the absolute best-for-you foods. The foods in white boxes are all pretty good (even if not ideal) to very good, but these are very best.*

Part 3: Lifestyle Audit

Whew! What a lot of foods to think about. Now you're almost done! The last section addresses your exercise habits and other health-related choices. Break out your pen and paper again, and get ready to write your answers! This is the third and final section of the Healthy U Check-Up.

1. If you have a routine exercise program, list each type of exercise that you do routinely, along with the number of times per week and the length of each session.

a. Include aerobic exercise (e.g. running, walking, biking, kaya-king, etc.), strength training (e.g. weight lifting, pushups, and sit-ups, etc.), and stretching and balance exercises (e.g. yoga).

b. Include activities that make you really work, such as playing tag with your kids or taking a long walk with your dog. Do not include regular household chores, such as vacuuming or dusting.

c. What upgrades are you willing to make to this program, starting today?

Example:
- Strength training with weights, 3x/week, 30 minutes each
- 2-mile walk with the dog, 6x/week, 30 minutes each
- Biking at the gym, 3x/week, 20 minutes each
- Stretching exercises, 5x/week, 10 minutes each

2. If you don't have a routine exercise program, what kind of exercise are you willing to start right now, how many days a week, and how long at one time? Remember, any exercise is better than no exercise, even 10 minutes! (This lifestyle audit is meant to help you track your overall progress. For guidelines on setting exercise goals, see Chapter 15. Please, always remember to check with your doctor before beginning or changing any exercise program!)

3. Do you work at a job that requires moderate to heavy physical activity? (In other words, something that makes you move around a lot, makes your heart beat faster, and makes you sweat.) What's that job, and how many hours a week do you physically work while on the job?

4. List prescription and non-prescription drugs (including supplements and herbal medications) you are taking, the dosage of each drug, and how many times a day you take it.

5. What medicines/supplements would you like to safely stop taking? Be specific. (And, of course, be sure to ask your health care practitioner to help you with this goal and to monitor you all along the way. Ask how much weight you would need to lose and/or what health milestones you would need to reach in order to safely reduce or eliminate each specific medication.)

Part 4: Get Intimate with Your Numbers

Write down your numbers. I'm guessing that most of you don't know these off the top of your head unless you've had a recent physical. So, if you're not sure, make an appointment to see your health provider. Tell him or her what you're doing and ask for help tracking these numbers. You may not be able to get your progress updates every month, but you should be able to get them at least twice a year.

Recording your numbers on a regular basis will help you track your tangible progress. *Seeing* your numbers go down from the efforts you make is a huge thrill, great self-reinforcement. It will spur you on to do even better! Make the effort as soon as possible to get your baseline (starting point) numbers.

Date   _____

Weight   _____

Height   _____

Age   _____

Body Mass Index (BMI)   _____

Blood Pressure   _____

Total Cholesterol   _____

Blood Glucose   _____

A1C   _____

Triglycerides   _____

Putting It All Together

Whoa, you finished! Now for the fun part. Let's talk about what all of these words and numbers mean.

The first section, called Soul Searching, facilitates self-discovery and written expression of your true feelings about your weight and body right now. It also helps you envision your ideal body-dream-come-true in one year, five years, and even ten years down the road in order to create doable one and five year goals for yourself. Tuck your written goals inside this book.

Then, when you take another look at this assessment in a month, three months, six months, a year, and beyond, you'll be able to re-read your original thoughts, desires, and specific goals to see where you started and how far you've come, which will reinforce your commitment to yourself. These goals represent the person you will become – if you *really* want it!

The second section, the Food/Beverage Audit, gives you a chart to track your progress at one month, three month and six month intervals. If you want to track for longer than that, photocopy the chart before you write on it and fill in dates for eight months, one year, and one and a half years.

On the chart, the very best-for-you foods are indicated by double asterisks (**), the better-for-you foods are listed in the white areas, and the worst-for-you foods are listed in the gray areas. This will all become much clearer after reading the next chapter. Each time you revisit this chart, you'll be amazed to see how your healthy food (white) numbers have gone up and your unhealthy food numbers (gray) have gone down. Over time, you may even notice that your natural preferences and tastes for healthy foods have increased. In fact, you'll actually find yourself eating lots more fresh fruit and vegetables and experiencing fewer cravings for meat, bread, cheese, sugar, salt, and even chocolate!

The third section, the Lifestyle Audit, helps you obtain baseline information about your exercise patterns and your medications, so you can set goals to upgrade both. Exercise is an important part of losing weight and building health. As your weight drops and your energy rises with the 10+10 for Life® program, you'll find yourself naturally gravitating more toward exercise. You'll finally feel more comfortable and capable of fully engaging in different activities, like walking, hiking, gardening, playing with your kids or grandkids, or swimming (in a bathing suit or – dare I say it? – even a two-piece for you gals).

Also, I encourage you to complete the fourth section with your doctor. Tell him or her about your new weight goals and lifestyle changes. Ask for help tracking the markers listed (blood pressure, blood work, BMI). It's exciting to watch these numbers improve as you eat better and better. I've worked with many people who have trimmed down to the point that their doctors safely reduce or eliminate medications. The investment of time and effort now can save your health, as well as big dollars spent for prescription and over-the-counter drugs.

The Next Steps into Your Pants

For now, we just have a baseline. To get to the next step, get your calendar out, and make three more dates with yourself:

1) One month from today   Date: _____

2) Three months from today   Date: _____

3) Six months from today   Date: _____

On each of these days, you will read what you wrote today and then retake the entire audit. Remember: you will need to write your answers to Parts 1 and 3 on separate paper. Part 2 – the big chart of different foods – was designed for you to write directly on the chart. However, you can photocopy it if you want to track yourself for longer than 6 months.

When consciously working toward a particular weight loss goal, charting your thoughts and progress along the way will help you stay on track. When you see yourself veering off track (which we all do), you will be so in tune and in touch that you'll quickly recognize the temporary detour and be able to jump right back on track. Charting takes a bit of time and effort, but the pay-off is huge – getting into those smaller pants.

As you progress through the program, you'll be able to peer into the mirror and feel the power of making more, better daily choices. As you retake the three parts of the Healthy U Check-up at the various time checkpoints, your improved numbers will fuel that drive and give you a way to record the strides you have made on your course to becoming a healthier, slimmer, happier YOU!

Now that you know your starting point and desired goals, let's move on to the rest of the book and learn how to get from here to there!

WHAT YOU NOW KNOW...

The answers to these questions:

- How do you **really** feel about yourself – inside and out?

- Where do you want to be one year, five years, and ten years from now?

- What foods do you eat?

- Do you exercise every day?

- Are you **really** ready to commit to YOU and getting into those pants?

Chapter 5

Add "10+10" to Wiggle Into Your Pants

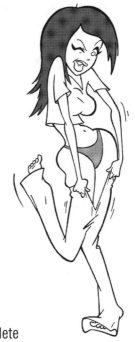

1. What is 10+10?

2. What to Eat: Feed vs. Deplete

3. How to Eat: The only three rules you'll ever have to know

   1. ADD   2. STOP   3. WIGGLE

WHAT IS 10+10?

Fruits and Vegetables Front and Center

L et's get down to the nitty-gritty and find out what 10+10 for Life® is all about. 10+10 is a practical eating plan that can help you reach your weight and health goals in reasonable time. Not only that, it does so without expensive, prepackaged diet foods, and without requiring you to count, measure, weigh, starve, deprive, feel guilty, or fuss ever again. This program is not meant to be a 3- or 6-

month quick-fix, weight-loss sprint, but rather a gentle, gradual lifestyle shift in thinking, eating habits, and your feelings about yourself.

10+10 for Life® was founded on the fundamental principle that whole, fresh fruits and vegetables are indisputably the best foods for human health and ideal weight and, therefore, deserve top priority at mealtime. However, we're so used to eating meals dominated by meat, cheese, milk, bread, and refined and processed foods it can be tricky to find room in our stomachs to eat enough fruits and vegetables.

10+10 is a simple solution to that challenge, which accomplishes the goals of enhancing health and lowering weight. The idea: eat the best-for-you foods first, namely fruits and vegetables, and eat the worst-for-you foods last. That way, you first fill up on those foods that boost your health and weight loss, without having to completely sacrifice your most beloved foods. In 10+10, your favorite food buddies are still "legal." It's just a matter of learning how and why you should shift their priority and eat them last – *after* you fill up on fruits and vegetables.

In other words, eat the good guys first and the bad guys last. Now doesn't that sound like a logical and doable strategy for losing weight while building up the health and energy that you crave?

10+10?

Just how many fruits and vegetables does 10+10 for Life® recommend?

You guessed it: 10 whole, fresh fruits + 10 different fresh vegetables!

How often? Every day (with a bit of wiggle room thrown in).

I'm sure that sounds like a lot of fruits and vegetables to eat in a day. So why do I recommend so many? Simple. It takes about that many fruits and vegetables to fill us up, especially after a lifetime of stuffing ourselves with heavy, dense foods like meat, cheese, and bread. And, as you may guess from your own experience with dieting, feeling full is absolutely critical for a program to work.

For Life?

As I pointed out in Chapter 4, this program is not a "diet." It's a lifestyle shift. That's why it's called 10+10 *for Life*®. And, for a program to work for a lifetime, a few other components are necessary, in addition to making sure you feel full and satisfied. A successful eating program must:

- Provide a complete array of life-supporting nutrients, including carbohydrates, protein, fats, vitamins, minerals, antioxidants, enzymes, phytochemicals, and all the discovered and yet to be discovered micronutrients.

- Be easy to understand and transition into from the exact place *you* are now.

- Be affordable and practical to incorporate into your life – for the rest of your life.

To address these needs, 10+10 for Life® is specifically designed to teach you first *what* to eat to obtain all the nutrients necessary for your health and energy. Then, it will teach you *how* to eat by following three easy to understand rules. Once you decide what's affordable and practical for you, you'll probably need to change some of your shopping, budgeting, and lifestyle habits to eat the 10+10 way.

However, as big or small as those changes may be, put them in perspective with the importance of your health. You're making an investment in both time and money to yourself and your family. And, you know what the big pay off is – finally getting into those pants!

With that said, let's move on to the fun part: What to eat and how to eat it!

WHAT TO EAT: FEED VS. DEPLETE

In our culture, we completely disconnect ourselves from the effects of what we eat. Food goes in, and food goes out. Most of us have little or no regard for what the food does to us in between. In other words, we don't make the association between the foods we choose to put into our bodies and how well we feel and move, our level of pep, the aging of our skin, the shine in our hair, the sparkle in our eyes, the bounce in our step, our level of productivity, our emotions, our self-esteem, our attitude, our clarity of thought, or our relationships. In fact, we typically eat for one purpose, and one purpose only – to satisfy and quiet the whines of those tiny, spoiled buds that sit on our tongues. (You thought I was going to say to fill us up, didn't you?)

There's one exception to the collective mindlessness of our food choices. And that's when we're counting calories or sizing up whether a food will add fat to our fat. But most of us leave out the most important question when counting calories: Which foods feed us, and which deplete us?

To be successful losing weight permanently, it's absolutely critical for you to get very clear *on the answer to this question*. The actual calorie count is less important than what nutrients those calories provide. And, that nutrient content is addressed by the concept of feed vs. deplete, the most critical concept in 10+10.

So, to make sure you understand it inside and out, we will go through a few steps.

First, I will explain the concept in-depth. Second, as you read through the book, the concepts of feeding and depleting will be woven into the explanations of different types of foods and food groups. Third, as you start practicing the 10+10 method for healthy eating and begin training your mind to automatically ask the question, "Does this food feed or deplete me?" the concepts you learn in this book will be reinforced.

However, just like the physical process of weight loss, the necessary learning that goes along with healthy eating takes time. So, don't be too hard on yourself if this concept doesn't solidify right away. I will make sure you get there.

Okay, here it goes.

Foods that feed us are critical for tip-top function and performance of our bodies at all times. Feed-me foods pack the biggest bang for our calorie buck. In other words, for each calorie we eat from a food that feeds us, we are receiving excellent nutrition with a wealth of macronutrients (carbohydrates, proteins, fats) and micronutrients (vitamins, minerals, antioxidants), enzymes, and fiber from which our bodies can pick and choose to fulfill their specific needs at any given moment. Feed-me foods prevent most of our chronic, degenerative, and killer diseases like many cancers, heart disease, type 2 diabetes, and stroke. It's no coincidence that these feed-me foods are also the foods that are absolutely critical for sustained weight loss.

On the other hand, foods that deplete us have far fewer nutrients per calorie. In fact, our bodies have to overwork to process and get rid of the bad stuff that comes in these deplete-me foods, whether it be fat, cholesterol, manmade chemicals, oils, salt, white sugar, or refined flours. And the extra fat and calories that come with these foods end up stored right where we don't want them – in our fat layers.

Here is a chart outlining the basic concepts behind foods that feed vs. foods that deplete:

FOODS THAT FEED	FOODS THAT DEPLETE
Contain	**Contain**
- Good carbohydrates, sourced by unrefined plant foods - Plenty of plant fats - Plenty of plant proteins - Vital micronutrients (vitamins and minerals) per calorie - A plethora of enzymes - Antioxidants that fight aging and abnormal cell growth - Lots of fiber - Low amounts of sodium found naturally in whole, plant foods - Relatively few calories	- Bad carbs: refined sugars and/or white flours - Liquid oils (yes, even olive oil) - Hydrogenated fats and/or trans fats - Animal fats - Animal proteins - Dietary cholesterol - White salt (sodium chloride – table, rock, or sea salt) - Chemicals, additives, preservatives
Don't Contain	**Don't Contain**
- Bad carbs: refined sugars or refined flours - Animal fats, trans fats, hydrogenated fats, or liquid oils - Animal proteins - Dietary cholesterol - White salt - Chemicals, additives, preservatives	- Enough or any good carbohydrates, sourced by unrefined plant foods - Enough or any micronutrients (vitamins, minerals) per calorie - Enough or any enzymes - Enough or any antioxidants - Enough or any fiber

Raise	Raise
- Energy levels - The will to exercise - Libido	- Body weight - Body mass index - Blood pressure - Cholesterol - Blood glucose (sugar in the blood) - Triglycerides (fat in the blood) - Risk of cancer, heart disease, stroke, type 2 diabetes and other diseases
Lower	**Lower**
- Body weight - Body mass index - Blood pressure - Cholesterol - Blood glucose (sugar in blood) - Triglycerides (fat in blood) - Risk of cancer, heart disease, stroke, type 2 diabetes, and other diseases	- Energy levels - The desire to exercise - Libido

Connecting, Choices, and Getting into Your Pants

Now that you know what feeding and depleting foods do, you can start to understand why you will be making certain food choices. After all, losing weight is all about choices. If you get more connected to the foods you eat, you'll begin the process of making more, better choices. It's as simple, and as complicated, as that.

And, if you continue to consciously make more, better choices then someday those choices will be programmed on auto-pilot and become easy to make. Trust me, I am traveling that same road. Better choices do become automatic, some sooner than others. It's such a relief to be free from food bondage, instead of thinking about food every waking minute.

To become more aware of the foods you eat, so you'll start making those better choices, I have a simple suggestion. Every time you eat something, say this to yourself: "Does this food feed me or deplete me?" And when I say every time, I mean every bite you put into your mouth. If you decide a particular food "feeds" you, congratulate yourself for making a wise food choice. If it "depletes" you, then it's up to you to recognize that fact and then make a decision whether or not you are going to eat it.

You are the master of your own choices and either the beneficiary or the slave of the consequences. Be aware of your choices and own them.

So now you know what feed-me foods offer and what deplete-me foods don't offer. But, unless you have a background in nutrition, you're probably still wondering, "What are the actual foods that feed me and what are the actual foods that deplete me?"

After a while, distinguishing the feed-me foods from the deplete-me foods will be easier for you. To get you started, I've included a chart with different kinds of foods, beverages, and snacks, listing foods that feed down to foods that deplete. It doesn't list everything. But, if you really have a question about a particular food or drink, you should be able to find something similar to it here.

The higher a box is in the chart, the more the foods/beverages in that box feed you, and the less they deplete you. 10+10 for Life® centers on the idea that at least eighty percent of your food should come from the top three boxes in this chart. The top box represents the best possible foods. The second box represents fairly healthy foods. The third represents transitional foods, that aren't horrible, but should be extremely limited. And the last box represents completely depleting, bad-for-you foods.

First Choice foods	
- Ideal feed-me foods. - Promote weight loss. - Fight diseases. - Boost health. - Foundation for 10+10.	- Raw, fresh vegetables - Whole, fresh fruits - Sprouts – alfalfa, mung, clover, broccoli, bean - Raw, unsalted nuts and seeds (limited amounts) - Fresh, homemade fruit and vegetable juices - Oil-, dairy-, sugar-, salt-, chemical-free salad dressings - Beverages: Water, non-caffeinated herbal teas
Second Choice foods	
- Very good feed-me foods. - Promote weight loss. - Fight diseases. - Boost health. - Eaten after ideal feed-me foods.	- Lightly cooked fresh vegetables, no salt, butter, margarine, or cheese - Frozen fresh fruits, no sugar - Heated frozen vegetables, no salt or added fat - Cooked fresh fruits, no sugar - Whole grains - brown rice, barley, whole oats, whole wheat couscous - Home-cooked dried beans - Oil-free, dairy-free salad dressings

Third Choice foods

- Fairly good choices.
- Feed us in some ways, deplete in others.
- "Transitional foods"
  – bridge from deplete-me foods to ideal feed-me foods.
- Not best choices
  – better than deplete-me foods in next two boxes.
	- Canned beans, no added fat or salt
	- 100% sprouted-grain bread
	- 100% whole grain bread
	- 100% whole wheat/corn tortilla shells
	- Dried fruit, no added sugar
	- Canned vegetables, no salt
	- Canned fruits, no sugar
	- Fat-free refried beans
	- Meat substitutes: tofu, soy, tempeh, seitan, minimal salt/chemicals/oils
	- Commercial, unsweetened 100% juice
	- Rice, soy, almond milk
	- Raw honey

Last Choice foods

- Bad-for-you, deplete-me foods. - Hinder weight loss. - Compromise health. - Drain energy. - Wiggle room (20%) foods. (Discussed in rule #3) Every bite, ask yourself, "Does this food feed me or deplete me?" Then decide whether to eat it or not. Remember, you don't have to "give up" anything on 10+10. You just have to shift your priorities and "add" the best-for-you foods!	- All meats: beef, poultry, pork, lamb, bison, seafood - All dairy products: milk, cheese, yogurt, butter, cream, ice cream, butter substitutes - Eggs - White flour products: breads, muffins, bagels, baked goodies - Boxed cereals - Refined sugars: white, brown, corn syrup, sucrose, lactose, fructose, dextrose, dextrin, cane juice, malt - Artificial sweeteners: aspartame, Splenda, stevia - Sugary desserts: cookies, cakes, doughnuts, pastries, pies - Candy (yes, even dark chocolate) - Trans fats/hydrogenated fats - Processed, clear liquid oils (even olive oil) - Oil-, dairy-based salad dressings - Deep fried: French fries, onion rings, fish, chicken - Processed and refined foods: white rice, frozen dinners, packaged diet foods, energy/protein/granola bars - Salty snacks: chips, pretzels, popcorn - Fast foods: burgers, fries, chicken, breakfast sandwiches, tacos, pop, milkshakes - Canned vegetables/beans with fat and/or salt - Roasted, salted nuts, nut mixes - Pizza - Beverages: alcohol, coffee (regular, decaffeinated), coffee drinks (mochas, lattes), caffeinated teas, soft drinks (diet, regular), protein/diet drinks, energy/sports drinks, store-bought juice with added sugar

This chart includes a wide spectrum of foods, as you can see. It's not all perfectly clear cut. Whether you're at home or making a decision in a restaurant, use your common sense and make the best possible choices. Very few people eat perfectly. However, the more "ideal" and "very good" feed-me foods you eat, the faster you will lose weight and get into those pants, and boost your health and energy besides.

My general rule of thumb for better choices is: "Raw is better than cooked, plant is better than animal, no oil is better than any oil."

As listed in this chart, consider substituting a healthier alternative for a popular (and worst) deplete-me food. Some alternatives are better than others.

Worst Foods	Better Choices
Pizza Delivery	Homemade pizza with whole wheat crust, soy cheese, and veggies
Hamburger	Veggie burger on whole wheat bun, tomato, lettuce, and sprouts
French fries	Baked potato strips
Beef taco	Black bean taco with guacamole, tomatoes, onions, jalapeños, lettuce wrapped in a whole wheat tortilla shell
Barbequed chicken	Grilled portabella mushroom and veggies
Stir-fried vegetables in oil	Stir-fried vegetables in water
Meat/dairy soup	Bean soup with veggies

Meat/dairy sandwich on brown-colored white bread	Avocado, veggie sandwich on 100% sprouted-grain bread
Hash browns fried in oil	Chopped potatoes steamed, then browned with water
Diet pop	Commercial or homemade fresh juices
Oil-based salad dressing	Water-based salad dressing
Milk shake	Fresh/frozen fruit smoothie with juice base
Mayonnaise spread	Hummus or avocado spread
Potato/butter/sour cream	Potato/pureed avocado/onions/tomato/cilantro
Roasted, salted almonds	Raw, unsalted almonds
Coffee	Grain coffee substitute, like Caffix or non-caffeinated, herbal tea
Dried cereal/cow's milk	Whole, cooked oats with raisins, fruit, rice milk, raw honey

Recap

Let's review. It's absolutely vital that you understand:

1. Certain foods feed, and certain foods deplete.

2. Foods that feed offer nutrients and promote health and weight loss. Foods that deplete offer extra calories and destroy health.

3. All foods fit somewhere on the spectrum between 100% feeding and 100% depleting.

4. Every time you take a bite, ask yourself. "Does this feed me or deplete me?" Then, make a conscious choice about whether to eat that bite.

5. There are healthier alternatives to almost all foods that deplete.

Now, with those concepts guiding your decisions about what to eat, let's get into the rules about how to eat.

HOW TO EAT: THE ONLY THREE RULES YOU'LL EVER HAVE TO KNOW

10+10 for Life® has only three rules: Add, Stop, and Wiggle. (Sounds like a catchy new dance, doesn't it?) If you follow these rules, you'll shed layers, inside and out, and greatly enhance your health.

Rule #1: ADD (10+10)

The first rule is to think about *adding* 10+10 to your day. The first thing on your mind, on your plate, and in your mouth at every meal, should be 10+10 (as in 10 whole fresh fruits and 10 different fresh vegetables.) And no, I don't mean that you're eating 10 fruits and 10 veggies at each meal. And yes, 10 seems like a high number. But, don't worry so much about the number. Ten is merely a benchmark, not a food law. When I walk you through your meals in the next three chapters, you'll see for yourself that reaching 10+10 is much easier than you think.

The bottom line is, each time you eat fill up on the best-for-you-foods first – fruits and vegetables. These foods *feed* you, remember? So, they need to be *added* at the beginning of each meal. And, you should eat them until you're really, truly full.

But, it's always important to allow yourself the freedom of choice to eat whatever foods you want if you're still hungry after you add 10+10. This freedom of choice is crucial. After all, what's the first thought that pops into your mind when you make the decision to lose weight? Do you moan and groan and think, "Okay, what am I going to 'have to' give up this time to get this weight off?"

And does that first hint of food-separation anxiety make that little-kid brat in you rear its ugly head and say, "Oh no, nope, no way, I'm not going to give THAT up. I'm gonna eat whatever I want"?

Or maybe that little-kid brat in you reluctantly concedes, "Okay, I'll give that up, but only for a month or three months or even a year or until I hit a certain weight, but I'm certainly not going to give that up forever. That's my favorite." So weight comes off while you sacrifice and stew. When the little-kid brat reclaims control, weight boomer-angs back on.

In 10+10 for Life®, if you follow the three simple rules, the brat disappears. You don't "have to" give up anything. Instead, you get to *add* to your food day. No more whining "poor me" even before you begin. With this food plan, you "get to" add for the purpose of sub-tracting, (weight, that is). Isn't thinking about what you "get to" add a refreshingly original way to think about food when you have sung the separation blues so many times before?

So, give yourself a psychological boost by thinking about all the foods you get to add. After you add these fresh fruits and vegetables, freedom is yours to eat the other stuff, if and only if you still have room!

Rule #2: STOP (Stop Eating When You're Full!)

The second rule is simple too. In fact, it's so simple that most people giggle when they hear it: STOP eating when you're full.

This may sound like a no-brainer, but most of us eat until our stomachs are overfull and over-distended. By that time, we have eaten too much food and too many calories. If you pay attention to your body's natural signals, your brain tells you that you are satisfied and full before your stomach screams at you and begs for mercy.

That satisfied, full feeling in your brain, so to speak, is a different feeling than that heavy feeling in your stomach you're used to. It takes time to distinguish the difference, but after you really pay attention to your body's smart, self-talk, you'll notice that, when you're eating, a switch flips in your brain, and your brain says, "Okay, I'm satisfied. I'm full. I've had enough." Your stomach will have a distinctly lighter feeling that will take time to get used to. But, after a while, you'll prefer the comfort of this lighter feeling to that over-full feeling you have grown accustomed to – the feeling that bogs you down and makes you want to curl up on the couch and take a nap. This lighter feeling is very, very different from being hungry.

I want you to be full. Truly and totally full. But then, when your brain speaks to you, do what you're told – STOP eating! Even if it's the best-for-you foods that you're leaving on your plate. It's more wasteful to put unneeded food into your body, which puts layers on your layers, than to put uneaten food down the garbage disposal. Garbage disposals are replaceable. You are not.

Rule #3: WIGGLE, if you must! (The 80/20 Rule)

The third and last rule is all about wiggle room. Let's face it right now. The instant you trap yourself in a restrictive food box of do's, and especially don'ts, you'll get obsessed with one thought: ESCAPE! After all your practice, you're a master escape artist. You know all the tricks.

Think about it. How many times in the past have you made a pact with yourself never, ever to eat certain foods again, and how many times did you break your pact, sometimes as soon as that same day? Probably every time, right? So don't make promises with yourself that you'll never keep. With 10+10, you don't "have to" give anything up.

This program is about teaching you the best way to eat and then giving you the freedom of choice. I trust you will make the right choices, most of the time, because you're a capable adult and care about yourself.

Build flexibility into your tailored-to-you eating plan from the very beginning. And know from the get-go that you will not be perfect, and you'll get off track, not just once but time and again. It's a given. So what? Just get back on track again the next meal, the next day, or the next week. The only slip up is to give up.

So how much wiggle room can you allow yourself and still lose weight?

To gauge your wiggle room, follow the "Casual/Dress-up Strategy" or the "80/20 Rule." Let's pretend you dress casually 80% of the time and that you dress up 20% of the time. Use that same 80/20 logic for your eating habits. On an average day when your environment is routine and under your complete control, consciously eat well by filling up on 10+10. Roughly 80% of the time. But when there's a special occasion, whether it's an anniversary, a neighborhood barbeque, dinner with guests, or you just want a change-up from the routine, eat whatever you want and enjoy it. Don't feel guilty. Do get back on track the next meal or day! For most of us, that's probably no more than 20% of the time. Interestingly enough, after a while, you'll find yourself naturally gravitating toward wiser, healthier choices, even on those "dress-up" occasions.

So the next time you choose to eat that chocolate birthday cake or traditional turkey dinner with all the trimmings, feel good about the fact that those foods are perfectly legal if they fall within that 20%. Wiggle room allows you the flexibility, self-kindness, and patience to stay on course for the long haul of your life.

WARNING! Be vigilant and very protective of your 80% territory and don't allow the 20% to creep in and take over. Sometimes the longer and/or more frequently you veer from 10+10, the more hooked you become in your old ways of eating, and the more difficult it is to get back on track.

The more fresh fruits and vegetables you eat every day, the more successful you will be at steady, consistent weight loss (2.5 pounds a month!) and ultimately getting into your pants. If you don't lose weight as quickly as you think you should, first make sure you are being reasonable with your goals, and then closely track exactly what you're eating. More than likely, you'll find that you are wiggling too much – eating too many deplete-me foods and not nearly enough feed-me foods. Be honest – you can't hide from yourself – your body shows all.

Recap

Be absolutely sure you're filling up at every meal, mostly on fresh, whole fruits and vegetables, then adding whole grains, beans, and whole breads **after** the vegetables. Finally, you can choose traditional meat and pasta dishes at the end of the meal, if you're still hungry. This method of eating automatically cuts calories and bad foods since you're first filling up on delicious, low-cal, good-for-you fresh foods.

Ultimately, you *will* succeed at losing weight *if* you fill up on the best-for-you foods.

But, losing weight is not about all-or-nothing, black-and-white success or failure. It's a process of making shifts and making more, better choices – every day. It's not about feeling hopeless or guilty or weak or dumb because you choose to eat something that you know isn't good for you. It's about giving yourself some wiggle room as you break through old habits while creating new, healthier habits. It's about feeling good about you. It's about your sheer determination and deep-down guts that make you to get up one more time than you fall. And, if you keep getting yourself up and back on track, you will, eventually, get into your pants.

As you're making your food choices, both good and bad, take responsibility, own your decisions, and keep the 10+10 mantra in the forefront of your mind: Add. Stop. And, wiggle, if you must!

WHAT YOU NOW KNOW...

- 10+10 for Life® means eating 10 whole, fresh fruits and 10 different, fresh vegetables every day.

- Which foods feed you and which foods deplete you.

- 10+10's three simple rules to get into your pants:

    1. **Add** and fill up on 10 fruits +10 vegetables every day.

    2. **Stop** eating when your brain tells you to.

    3. **Wiggle**, if you must. Watch it! No more than 20% of the time.

Chapter 6

Breakfast: Morning Delights for Skinnier Pants

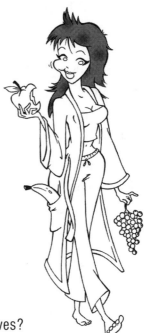

What's up for breakfast?

- What are your morning faves?

- What are some better choices?

- What "Big Buts" are blocking your way?

Rise and shine. It's breakfast time! We've taken a look at the concepts and guidelines of 10+10. Now, let's get specific, beginning with the foods that start your day.

First, we'll discuss your breakfast personality and your traditional breakfast favorites. Then we'll open your eyes to another option – one that fits 10+10 for Life®, aimed at helping you reach your own personal weight-loss and health goals. Finally, we'll peel back some common breakfast misconceptions and expose your morning "big buts" that keep you out of those pants.

WHAT ARE YOUR MORNING FAVES?

If you're like most Americans, you've probably developed a pretty distinct breakfast personality. Maybe you hit the snooze button three times, roll out of bed at the very last minute, and jam a piece of toast and a cup of coffee into your mouth as you scurry out the door. Or you may revel in the quiet, early-morning hours, slow-to-wake up before enjoying a leisurely breakfast with traditional favorites. Perhaps you have a long commute to work and eat on the go after a stop at the doughnut shop or your favorite fast food place. Maybe you just aren't hungry in the morning, or you're "saving" calories and skip breakfast altogether. Or, you might have a breakfast personality different than any of these.

Whichever breakfast personality is yours, it's important to remember that breakfast is a big chunk of your eating day, and your life for that matter – one-third to be exact. Every morning you have the opportunity to get off on either the right foot, nourishing your body with the best-for-you-foods, or the wrong foot, sabotaging your health and weight goals with bad-for-you-foods. So, let's talk about some of the choices you can make.

Which Favorites Fit 10+10?

Regardless of your breakfast personality, most of us love to eat the familiar American breakfast foods we grew up with: dried, boxed cereals with cows' milk (that perfect food for baby cows), instant oats with brown sugar, eggs, yogurt, toast, butter, jam, bagels, muffins, bacon, sausage, ham, pancakes, waffles, syrup, hash browns, doughnuts, and sweet pastries. We wash it all down with orange juice and America's pick-me-up and drop-me-down morning sweetheart, coffee (or better yet, a mocha-latte with whipped cream).

So, let's apply what we learned in the last chapter to the foods listed in the above paragraph to try to figure out which of these favorites fit into 10+10. Read through the list again and try to determine which of those foods feed you and which deplete you. If you need a minute to flip back a few pages and check the Feed vs. Deplete Chart of Foods, go ahead!

Now, let's see how you did. When going down the list, did you get hit by an ah-ha moment – like maybe none of your morning favorites make the top 10+10 hits? If you did, you are not alone. The process of realizing what you are eating and how it affects you can be shocking the first time you start to really apply it to yourself. It might seem like all the foods you like are bad-for-you.

Are there any foods on the list that feed you? The only one here with potential is orange juice. And only if it's freshly made, with no added sugars or preservatives.

All the rest of the foods deplete you.

But remember, if your breakfast favorites deplete you, you don't have to part with them forever. The choices about what to eat are always yours. If you feel like eating eggs, bacon, and coffee one morning, you have your wiggle room, if you must! But be aware that, when you use that wiggle room, you are depleting yourself. Make sure that most of your choices (at least 80%) are getting you closer to stepping into those pants.

Now that we've talked about traditional breakfast foods, let's talk about a new way to approach the first meal of the day.

WHAT ARE SOME BETTER CHOICES?

Allow me to help you gently climb out of the cardboard breakfast box and slowly tippy-toe into a foreign land of fruit and plenty. Open your mind and s-t-r-e-t-c-h your breakfast thinking. If what you're used to eating for breakfast doesn't feed you, then which foods do?

The answer: whole, fresh fruits, of course. Fresh fruits constitute perfect breakfast choices, by feeding, not depleting. Fruits are power-packed with disease-preventing and life-supporting carbohydrates (the good ones), proteins (yes, fruits have proteins), fats (and, yes, they even have fats), vitamins, minerals, antioxidants, phytochemicals, micronutrients, enzymes, water, and fiber. Some of the best nutrition for your calorie buck. And, lucky us, in this bountiful country of ours, we have plenty from which to choose all year long.

No, 10+10 breakfasts are not like the big sit-down meal we grew up with. And, it's not like the grab-as-fast-as-you-can breakfast we raised our kids on. The idea here is somewhere in the middle. You eat a lot of food, but you graze on it all morning long. It is fast, as there is little to no preparation. You could start off with a couple of bananas and a few handfuls of strawberries and blueberries, then move on to two oranges and a nectarine, and finish later in your morning with an apple and a big bunch of grapes.

The idea is to eat as many as, or even more than, 10 whole, fresh fruits between the time you wake up, and about an hour before lunch. And, as I said before, 10 is not a magic number. If you are truly full with 5 fruits, stop there. If you make it to 15, that's fine too. And you don't have to (and shouldn't) eat your fruits all at once.

Remember: Add, Stop, and Wiggle!

First, you add fruit until you're full. Graze throughout the morning and, each time you start to feel hungry, have some of whatever fruit you have available that morning. Then, each time you are satisfied stop eating. You should do this throughout the morning.

And, as I mentioned before, if you need, or want rather, a dough-nut and coffee, or some pancakes and eggs, or even a big Sunday brunch, go for it and enjoy it. Get back into 10+10 as soon as possible, whether by lunchtime, the next day, or the next week. The more often you follow 10+10, the more constant your weight loss will be.

Now that I've told you to pretty much scrap your breakfast faves and try to get by on fruit alone, are you scared?

I know that eating only fresh fruit in the morning may be a big leap for you. Let me try to ease some of your fears.

First, don't be afraid you'll be hungry. I want you to feel full – all morning! Your body talks to you. Pay attention to it and listen to your hunger drive. Eat fruit throughout the morning whenever you feel hungry. My clients are often shocked when they find out for themselves that they can actually fill up on fruit, often a brand new experience for them. And, trust me, it takes way more than that one apple a day we grew up with.

Second, stop being afraid of giving up your favorite foods. That 20% wiggle room is vital to the success of this program – to let your-self wiggle, if you must. And, interestingly enough, when you flex your options and keep coming back to the 10+10 way of eating, you will, eventually, start to find yourself gravitating naturally toward healthier choices and wiggling less.

Third, don't worry about whether planning and preparing your breakfast will take extra time. Fruits are the ultimate fast foods: wash or peel, open mouth, insert, bite down, and chew. I mean, you *can* make more work for yourself and make fruit salads with chopping, peeling, dicing and slicing. But what's the point? Why do we women insist on making complicated out of simple, followed by complaining about the extra work we create for ourselves? Sometimes I just don't get us, do you?

Not only are fruits easy to grab fast, they are easily transportable. Bring them with you in the car, to work, on trips, and for any extra curricular activities. I go everywhere with my "have-fruit-will-travel" container, complete with a plastic bag for the peels, pits, and cores, and a few napkins for piggy me.

And fourth, don't be daunted by trying to figure out how many serving sizes come with each fruit and what, exactly, constitutes a "whole" fruit. I will explain it all, in detail.

What Does the "Whole" in Fruit Mean?

Don't worry, this concept is not tricky. Don't make it more complicated than it actually is! Usually, but not always, "whole" translates to "one whole" fresh fruit as in one apple, one orange, one peach, one plum, one nectarine, one grapefruit, one pear, one mango, or one banana. And, you can eat as many of one fruit as you want. In other words, if you really want a 10-orange morning, go for it. Most likely, though, it will be a mix of fruits, as in two apples, three oranges, one mango, a bunch of grapes, and two bananas. Just think of all your ex-diets and laugh. No more half bananas for you. Be honest – did that half banana ever make sense to you? You are now free to eat the whole thing and – drum roll please – even two or three if you'd like! Now, if that doesn't shock the pants off you, nothing else in this program will!

Of course not all fruits fall into the "one whole" fruit rule. Larger fruits, as in melons or pineapples, can be counted for more than "one whole" fruit depending on the size. A cantaloupe, for example, can count for about three whole fruits.

On the other hand, about two handfuls of very small fruits, as in grapes, cherries, or berries, count as one whole fruit in the 10 fruit count. Pleeease don't count the number of grapes or berries. Use your common sense, and don't get stuck on the small stuff – like exactly how many "whole" fruits make up one watermelon. Eat until you're full of watermelon. The fullness is what matters. The number is just a fill-you-up guideline.

The point is, graze all morning on enough fresh fruit to satisfy your hunger drive. Then stop eating when you're full. It's that simple.

Morning Grazing Ideas

To give you an idea of a 10+10 morning, here's one of mine during the work week.

I get up at 4:45 am, wash my fruit, work out, and then start grazing at my office right before I see my first patients at 7:30. In fact, I start munching away the minute I get into my car after exercising. I'm hungry by then! I usually start with about three bananas (no, I'm not kidding), a crunchy apple, a bunch of grapes and, depending on the season, an orange or two, or maybe a nectarine and a plum. (How about it? Do you think that amount of fruit could fill you up, too?)

Throughout the morning, I fit in the rest of my 10, and often eat even more. Here are typical fruits you could choose, depending on the season and availability. You're certainly not limited to the fresh fruits on this list. Select those you enjoy.

Apples

Apricots

Bananas

Berries (count two large handfuls as one whole fruit)

Cantaloupe (count one whole cantaloupe as approximately three whole fruits – I often eat a whole one in one sitting!)

Fresh Figs (not dried)

Grapefruits

Grapes (count a big bunch as one whole fruit)

Guava

Kiwis

Mangoes

Nectarines

Oranges

Papayas

Peaches

Pears

Persimmons

Plums

Pineapple (count one whole pineapple as approximately 4 whole fruits)

Pomegranates

Pomelos

Starfruit

Tangerines

Ugly Fruit

If you haven't tried all the fruits on this list, expect a delightful treat. Just think about how many new foods you will get to add to your life with 10+10.

Toots with Fruits

However much you may be enjoying your fruit, I recommend that you stop eating fruit about one hour before lunch. While not a law, it's a good idea to put a little time between fruits and your noontime foods because fruits can cause other foods to ferment in your digestive system. And fermentation spells G-A-S. If you think that fruit causes you gas, don't mix fruits with other foods, and see if that helps.

WHAT "BIG BUTS" ARE BLOCKING YOUR WAY?

About this time I think I hear some mental rumblings out there that could ignite into an uproar of protests. I believe the rumblings all start with...but, but, but....

Let's bust through those "big buts," one at a time, so they no longer can keep you out of those pants.

"But, but, but...I'm not hungry in the morning."

If you aren't hungry in the morning, you are not alone. Have you ever wondered why you have no appetite first thing when you probably haven't eaten for over eight hours? You wouldn't want to go eight hours or more during the day without eating something, yet your stomach turns its nose up to breakfast.

Here's why: To process food, your body goes through three basic cycles: digestion from noon to 8:00 p.m., absorption from 8:00 p.m. to 4:00 a.m., and elimination from 4:00 a.m. to noon.

Skipping over the first two cycles, let's highlight the final cycle – the elimination cycle, which hits us in the morning, the body's natural time to get rid of waste. During the time when your body is working hard to clean itself out, there's less available energy to digest newly added food. The result: little or no hunger in the morning. This natural lack of hunger is compounded by your habit of not eating. Habits die hard!

Even if you fit into this "not hungry" category, try eating fruits as suggested in 10+10. Fruits are the easiest foods to digest, so eating them during the elimination phase makes sense. It's easier on your body. You may be delighted by how your body enjoys light, nutritious foods in the morning, and how easy it is to break your habits when your body is happy.

"But, but, but...I get fewer calories going without."

Although you may think skipping breakfast "saves" you calories, by the end of the day you are probably packing in more calories than if you ate breakfast, especially one consisting of whole fruits. The problem with skipping breakfast is that your body tends to get too hungry, resulting in overeating later in the day. Also, cravings often intensify because you aren't getting enough nutrition in a timely manner. Cravings hold you hostage to uncontrollable urges that drive you to binge and overeat the wrong kinds of foods and pseudo-foods that pile on excess calories that are empty of nutrients, and are overloaded with sugar, salt, cholesterol, fat, oils, and chemicals.

"But, but, but...I have to eat a big breakfast."

You are going to eat a big breakfast.

But not like the ones you're used to. Big breakfasts with typical American foods load you with fat, sugar, and calories, and bog you down with more weight. That is why, as we discussed, these foods deplete you. Even if you are one of those people who likes to eat a big breakfast so you don't have to eat again until noon, you may find that you actually like the way the lightness of fruit makes you feel instead of that full, sluggish feeling in your stomach. You don't have to feel heavy to feel full. The trick is to add enough fruits throughout the morning to fill you up and keep your hunger drive satisfied. This is very important.

"But, but, but...I can't get full on just fruit."

Oh, yes, you can! I have worked with hundreds of people (myself included) who have said the very same thing and have shocked and delighted themselves when they discovered they can and do get full on fruit – when they eat enough of it. We're just not pre-programmed to eat enough of it. Go ahead, try it and see for yourself. It's the easiest part of your food day.

"But, but, but...I work – I just don't have time to eat that much fruit."

I find that if you get your intentions and goals clear and wrap your brain around grazing on fresh fruit, then most people can carve out the time to slip in enough fruit throughout the morning to keep them satisfied and full.

However, if you are one of those people who works at a job that offers no breaks for four hours straight, you will have to use your common sense in adapting your eating habits to accommodate your job. You may want to eat more dense fruits that contain less water, like bananas. They tend to stick with you longer. Or you could eat a satisfying bowl of oatmeal with fresh fruit as a second choice to fruit on the mornings you have to work.

But if your workplace allows employees to take breaks for things like smoking and using the bathroom, why not try to take a fruit break. It only takes a moment to throw a handful of pre-washed grapes into your mouth, or to open your mouth, bite down, and chew pieces of an apple on your way to and from the bathroom. This is exactly what I do between patients during my busy day-to-day practice.

"But, but, but...I don't have time to shop for fresh fruits so many times a week."

Sorry. I don't buy it. Our modern day provides modern conveniences – like refrigerators. I find that shopping twice a week for fresh fruits is plenty. Not only that, I spend very little time in the store because I visit only the produce section, and I know exactly what I want and its location. In and out, lickety-split. If you still think it takes too much time, say this to yourself: shopping for fruits and vegetables doesn't take time, it gives me time when it counts – at the end of my life.

"But, but, but...fresh fruit is too expensive."

It's funny how we're willing to pay for meats, cheeses, doughnuts, processed foods, pizza, desserts, diet pops, and chips, not to mention eating out several times a week, expensive prepackaged diet foods, or $4-a-day coffee mochas, yet we flinch at investing in our own health and successful weight loss with nature's best – fruits and vegetables.

Not only that, eating correctly by filling up on the 10+10 can save you big dollars in doctor bills, medications, and lost wages from not being able to work due to poor health.

"But, but, but...I get bored with so little variety."

Our country blesses us with a huge variety of fruits, as well as vegetables, with dozens of different flavors and textures, almost all year long. Be patient. It takes time to retrain your taste buds, spoiled by a lifetime of sugar, salt, and artificial flavorings. But they and you are trainable and can be totally satisfied by the natural sweetness and flavors of fruits. I've seen it time and time again. Patience and time are the keys.

In the meantime, it's interesting how we cry "boring" with fruits or vegetables, yet most Americans eat only about fifteen different foods from the standard American fare anyway and never get bored. I've never ever heard anyone whine about getting bored with pizza, burgers, steaks, chicken and gravy, ham and cheese sandwiches, chocolate, or coffee.

Boring just may have everything to do with habit, rather than how much variety we get from our foods.

"But, but, but...I'm hypoglycemic."

You may think that you have hypoglycemia, or low blood sugar, that causes you to get light-headed and jittery when you eat only fruit. Many people, with or without symptoms of hypoglycemia, get light-headed, not because they are eating too much fruit, but because they are eating too little fruit. If you eat with enough quantity and frequency to fill you up and satisfy your hunger drive, lightheadedness, along with hypoglycemia, can magically disappear. Any of us can get light-headed and jittery if we don't eat enough food and go too long between meals. But, as always, if you do have a medical condition like this, talk to your doctor about your new eating plan, and let him or her answer your questions and help you make the transition safely.

"But, but, but...fruit has too much sugar."

Somewhere along the way we started confusing our dietary "sugars." Without a doubt, refined sugar is one of the top bad guys. However, sugars from whole, fresh fruits and refined white sugar are totally different animals.

I will discuss this more in depth in a later chapter. To put it very simply for now, whole, fresh fruits and vegetables, our best sources of unrefined carbohydrates, are transformed by the body into glucose. Glucose is the fuel that provides the body with the energy that keeps us alive and fully charged. In fact, our brains run primarily on glucose alone. The energy we get today is provided by the fruits and vegetables we ate yesterday, not the meats, cheeses, milk, white bread, or protein bars we eat today.

"But, but, but...what about diabetes and fruit?"

A few conditions warrant caution when changing your diet to include more fruits. Diabetes type 1 and type 2 are two such conditions.

Before you begin any dietary changes, ask your doctor to help you monitor your blood glucose and diabetes. Make sure you feel comfortable testing yourself and that you understand all of the warning signs that your body will give you when your blood sugar falls below or rises above acceptable levels.

For type 2 diabetics especially, fruits can be an important part of losing the weight you need to reverse the disease. If you have type 1, you may be able to tolerate eating more fruit. Then again, maybe not.

If you have diabetes and don't feel that eating fruit all morning works for you, (or even if you don't have diabetes), then, as mentioned, a good second choice for morning nutrition is cooked, whole oats, ideally mixed with fruit and soy or rice milk. Do what you can to make healthy choices.

ONE-THIRD DOWN, ONLY TWO-THIRDS TO GO...

Way to go! You've already grazed your way through the first third of your day, and it wasn't even that hard. Talk about fast food. How much faster and simpler can you get than wash, open mouth, bite down, and chew? And the good news is, lunch is coming right up, and that's simple, too. The truth is, as you become more and more familiar with 10+10, you'll find the simpler choices usually offer the most nutrition for the calorie buck. And, the more simple choices you make, the more quickly you'll ease yourself into those pants.

WHAT YOU NOW KNOW...

- Which deplete-me foods you used to choose for breakfast.
- The ideal morning delights: up to 10 whole, fresh fruits.
- Which big breakfast buts keep you out of your pants.

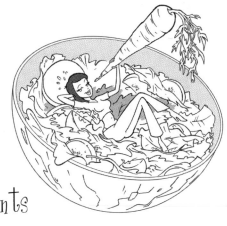

Chapter 7

The Nooner –
Slipping OUT of Your Pants

What's up for lunch?

- What are your noontime faves?

- What are some better choices?

- What "Big Buts" block your way?

N ow that you've jumpstarted your day the 10+10 way with
whole, fresh fruits, let's give your rusty, old Cinderella lunchbox a shake and shift your attention to the brilliant Technicolor
of the ideal 10+10 nooner.

WHAT ARE YOUR NOONTIME FAVES?

A sandwich kind of love affair

If we take a peek inside your lunchbox, I bet we all know what's inside.
Ah, yes, a sandwich, of course. We Americans looooooove sandwiches
(myself included). Even today, after years of not indulging in the beloved American meat and cheese sandwich, my mouth still waters just

thinking about them. And, I don't love just one or two kinds of sandwiches. I love all kinds of sandwiches with all kinds of favorite delights stacked between all kinds of breads. You name it, I love it. And you probably do, too.

Start with the bread – wheat, rye, pumpernickel, multi-grained, sourdough, French – and slather the slices or rolls with good, ole' fashion REAL Hellmann's mayonnaise. Then build the layers from the bottom up, first the meat, almost any kind will do: turkey, chicken, roast beef, ham, bologna, or liverwurst.

Then add the layer of cheese, and oh so many delectable choices: extra sharp, sharp, medium and mild cheddar, havarti, jack, Swiss, mozzarella, and American, to name only a few. Last, throw on the extras, like lettuce, tomatoes, pickles, and onions. Top it off with that luscious second slice of bread, and voila! One bite and I'm in sandwich heaven.

For a bit of variety, there's always tuna, egg salad, cream cheese and olives, scrambled eggs, BLT, and toasted cheese, not to mention the meatloaf, meatballs, or steak left over from the night before. Oh, and we mustn't forget the all-American standby, almost a food group in its own right for every kid or kid-at-heart – peanut butter and jelly.

Why are sandwiches so popular and irresistible? Simple. They taste great, fill us up, thrown together in a snap, and are eaten quickly with a no-fuss clean up. But more than that, they've have been a hit on the noontime parade from the time we abandoned the bottle. They are deeply etched into the memory banks of our senses – taste, smell, touch, sight – and are directly linked to persnickety taste buds and that warm and fuzzy center of our brains.

Thinking beyond your best buds for a minute, quickly peruse the lunch menu in your mind – sandwiches, subs, meat, creamy soups, burgers, shakes, hot dogs, chips, French fries, pizza, tacos, fried chicken, fried fish, tacos, combo-salads, like potato, macaroni, 3-bean, diet soda, sugary drinks, cookies, and maybe even a green-leafy, vegetable salad.

Starting off with that same question we asked at breakfast to find the best-for-you noontime foods, let's look through all the foods I just named – all the ones in the last five paragraphs, starting with breads. Now, which of the foods listed feed you and which ones deplete you?

Let's start with feed-me foods. What did you come up with? I found a few. If you used 100% whole wheat or sprouted-grain bread in your sandwich, that's okay. Not perfect, but reasonable. The green salad mentioned (minus any oil-based dressing) was great. So were the single slice of tomato and the lonely lettuce leaf sitting inside a sandwich. And then, if I really scratch around, I might be able to make a case for the cooked-to-death vegetables in the creamy soup (if there was no cream), the potatoes in the potato salad (if there was no mayo), and the canned beans in the bean salad (nix the oil).

All of the other foods deplete you. (Did you get that ah-ha! moment again?)

So, I'd like to have a discussion about the good-for-you foods here. But, come on, who can get full and satisfied from a piece of bread, tomato slice, piece of lettuce, and small salad with no dressing? Let's talk about some feed-me foods with real substance and leave the depleting foods in the background where they belong.

WHAT ARE BETTER CHOICES?

Well, I'll give you a big hint. 10+10 stands for 10 fresh, whole fruits, and 10 different, raw veggies, and we fit our 10 fruits into breakfast. So, what's left?

10, count 'em 10 – fresh, raw, colorful, delicious vegetables. Eat them in a salad. Eat them whole like your fruits. Cut them up into squares and eat them with a fork. My preferred way to eat vegetables is in a salad. Just make sure you eat enough to fill you up!

The process of transitioning from super-filling sandwiches, or any of your other noontime celebrities, to lighter, healthier 10+10 salads may be a huge stretch for you, just like eating fruits only in the morning. It certainly was for me.

In fact, at one time I didn't think I could live without sandwiches. After all, what's left to eat for lunch if there are no sandwiches? However, gradually, almost without my realizing it, my love for green-leafy, vegetable salads grew while my lifelong lust for sandwiches fizzled, although my memory still flirts. Now, I feel cheated if I don't get my large, vegetable salad for lunch. With time, persistence, and lots of little, detour bunny trails along the way, tastes do change. Ignored, even disliked, foods can grow into favored, number one choices.

But back to the star of your show – you. Does that mean you have to eat exactly like me and ban your best buds for life? Not at all. No need for melodramatic "poor-me" sacrifices here. There's always that wiggle room, if you must! And, besides that, there exist better-for-you building blocks to make better-for-you sandwiches. We'll get to that. For now, let's find out why salads, if dressed appropriately, show-off a perfect "10" for the three 10+10 rules.

1. ADD 10

Add and fill up on green-leafy, vegetable salads for your 10+10 nooner. Remember, 10+10 is about adding, not giving up. So, let's add lots of green and rainbow colors, chock full of the best nutrition, to make you shine from the inside out and shed the weight.

Along with fruit, raw vegetables are the foundational foods upon which 10+10 was created and built. In this culture, salads just happen to be the tastiest, most streamlined, interesting way of throwing together a bunch of raw vegetables to create one appetizing and energizing lunch. Munching on carrot and celery sticks alone sounds neither appealing, filling, nor practical. You'd be munching all day and still be scavenging for more food.

By filling up on the perfect size salad for you with 10 different vegetables, it's only noonish, and you've already hit the 10+10 jackpot – 10 different vegetables and close to 10 fresh fruits, depending how many you ate during your morning grazing.

But can adding salads for lunch actually satisfy and fill you? Absolutely! Diving into a large, colorful vegetable salad bursting with many different flavors, colors, and textures can be both satisfying and filling – *if* you eat enough of it. And that's the trick. You must eat enough of your mixed-up, raw friends, or too many of those sneaky not-so-good-for-you foods fly into your open-like-a-baby-bird mouth.

2. STOP eating when full.

When you follow the first rule in 10+10 by adding and filling up on salad, the second 10+10 rule becomes automatic: stop eating when you're full!

One of the beauties of eating 10+10 salads for lunch is that you automatically stop eating when you're full. After all, can you remember the last time you ate too much vegetable salad? Just like fruit, that has probably never happened. And, no, it's not because salads are less delicious or you get 'sick' of eating them. It's because the usual foods you eat – laced with sugar, salt, fats, and artificial flavors, trick your brain into eating more. It's like any other addiction. After all, how many times have you had, say, a plate of pasta at a restaurant, or a piece of chocolate cake, and been totally stuffed, to the point where you put your fork down and say, "enough." And then, how many times have you picked up that fork again and taken "just one more bite" and then another, and then another, even though you were completely full?

No question. Foods are addictive, especially the ones, or some variation thereof, that we learned to love as tots. One of the biggest roadblocks preventing you from those pants is the ability to stop eating when full. It's easy with vegetable salads. When your brain tells you to stop eating, what do you do? You stop eating. And how many calories were in all those vegetables? Maybe 200 (without avocado or oil dressing) and you are *full!* It's not about self-control. It's about auto-stop. Fill up on the best-for-you foods, and you automatically stop eating. How perfect is that?

3. WIGGLE! (if you must!)

But of course there's always room for that wiggle (if you must!). When you go out to lunch with a friend, attend a Red Hatter, get together with your favorite group, or you just want a change-up from salads or other feed-me nooners, you're free to eat whatever you want. But, remember, be possessive of that 80% territory reserved for 10+10 foods. Don't allow other foods to creep in from their designated 20%.

Eating in the Raw

Why not cooked vegetables? What's so great about eating in the raw? When nature's best is raw, whole, unaltered, unadulterated, unprocessed, unrefined, and un-messed-with-in-any-way, it provides human beings with all the health-building nutrition they need to survive and thrive throughout a long lifetime. Sad, but true, most of us survive and maybe even thrive when we're younger, but we certainly don't thrive into our later years, if we actually survive that long.

Cooked vegetables and fruits, although an obvious better choice than most other foods, concede first place to their raw food champs. Cooking completely wipes out all enzymes needed for every single chemical reaction in your body, from the blinking of your eyelids, to the efficient processing of fat and calories, to an inkling of a thought. Cooking destroys most water-soluble vitamins, and minerals are denatured (made into different molecular shapes), devaluing their worth as well. Heat even breaks down the all-important fiber in fruits and vegetables, making it less effective than in its raw counterparts.

Because our raw health heroes and weight warriors are so essential to our very survival, raw fruits and vegetables were created with a wide spectrum of different tastes, colors, shapes, sizes, textures, and flavors, nature's way of enticing us humans to eat them.

Yet, nature-in-the-raw is not just another pretty face with substance. She's also an easy pick-up in our modern, convenient world. You drive to the local grocery store twice a week, push a cart, fill the cart with raw beauties, and bring them home. Then you wash, chop if necessary, open mouth, insert, and chew. How much easier can you get? You don't even have to cook! Now that's complete freedom from food frenzy.

And, the very best part of all, raw vegetables are naturally low in calories. When it comes to calories, I compare eating vegetables to eating air. That means you can *and must* eat as much as you want! After over eating, restricting, starving, bingeing, and fretting about food for much of your life, can you even imagine what it would be like to be free to eat as much as you want whenever you want?

Well, imagine no more. Your fairy-tale dream to eat to your body's complete and utter delight just came true – as long as you eat the feed-me foods. Check out these calorie counts for raw foods:

4 cups of Romaine lettuce: 32 calories

2 cups of cucumbers: 28 calories

1 tomato: 24 calories

2 cups of red cabbage: 40 calories

2 cups of spinach: 24 calories

1 cup of broccoli: 24 calories

1 cup of cauliflower: 24 calories

1 cup of red or green pepper: 24 calories

½ cup onion: 27 calories

Grand total for way more than you can eat in one sitting: only 247 calories!

Compare those numbers to one McDonald's measly hamburger, not even a cheeseburger. Without the fries, without the toppings. Just that tiny little burger and bun: 300 calories. Now, to eat enough to fill you up at McD's, let's add medium fries, and, say, a small soda. Medium fries: 380 cal (yes, more than the burger). Small soda: 150.

So you can spend 830 calories having a meal at McDonalds and get, let's see, how many enzymes, antioxidants and good carbs? That's right – zero. There's nothing nutritious, fresh, or otherwise healthy about this meal. Nothing. You have eaten almost half of the calories that most women need per day. And I'll bet in another hour you'll be hungry again.

Or, you can spend 247 calories stuffing yourself with vital nutrients and eat as much as you want later when you get hungry.

The bottom line is this: do you *really* want to lose weight and keep it off and build your health at the same time? Of course you do. That's why you're here and making the effort to learn a new way of eating. As I've said before, and I'll say again, in order to slip easily in and out of those pants, center your food-life around the very best-for-you foods – fresh, raw fruits and vegetables.

"But, but, but…." I can read your mind. Hang on, we'll get to your "big buts" in a minute. For right now, let's dive head-first into that salad.

The 10+10 in 10 Chop Salad

I want to share with you a basic salad I like to make every day. I call it the 10+10 in 10 Chop Salad. The last 10 stands for the 10 minutes required to make this salad.

Start with a large base of lettuce, enough to fill you up. How large is large? Again, play around with this. It won't take you long to know how much salad will fill you up and keep you full for at least two hours. To give you an idea, when I make enough salad for just myself, I fill up the largest Pyrex bowl of the four stacked glass bowls we all use in the kitchen. That's about one whole head of lettuce, depending on the size. I know. I know. It's hard to believe I can eat all that salad, but it's true, and I have lots of witnesses who will vouch for me. Would this much salad fill you up as well? My guess? Yes. But find out for yourself how much salad is right for you.

When it comes to choosing the best-for-you lettuce, think green, the greener the better. Romaine, green-leaf, red-leaf, oak-leaf, butter or bib, spinach, endive, radicchio, and baby greens are good choices. Iceberg (which my kids call "candy" lettuce) is a less ideal choice, because it's less green, meaning it contains fewer nutrients than the greener lettuces and vegetables. But, if iceberg is what will get you to eat salads, go for it. Then slowly start to introduce other varieties.

After you choose your lettuce, add enough other vegetables to the lettuce to reach 10 or so. Add as many different colors as possible to ensure you get all of the micronutrients (vitamins, minerals, enzymes, phytochemicals, antioxidants, etc.) I count every vegetable as one vegetable. If I add two different kinds of lettuce, I count them as two different vegetables. If I add two kinds of sprouts, I count them as two vegetables. As you can see, it doesn't take long to reach the goal of 10 vegetables in your salad. Add enough of each vegetable so that, when you toss it around, you can see them all. It should look like a big rainbow of colors.

Below is a simple recipe for my 10+10 in 10 Chop Salad. Make changes and substitutions wherever you'd like. This is your lunch, not mine.

As a side note, let's not get overly picky. It's true, some of the foods we may think of as vegetables are technically fruits, like avocados, cucumbers, and tomatoes, but I still count them as vegetables for the 10-vegetable count. Again, filling up on fruits and vegetables is what's important, not debating over the category they fall into.

One more thing, although I use measurements in the recipe to give you an idea of quantities, I never actually measure the vegetables. I just make sure I add 10 different ones and that I can see them all when I mix the salad around. (In other words, just one baby carrot would get hidden). Use common sense to find your portions. Eat whatever quantity of each vegetable you want to each day. Forget measuring. Just throw a bunch of vegetables together into a bowl and eat them until you're full. Simple! One big salad fills you and satisfies your hunger drive.

If you have pre-washed the greens and have the right tools on hand, with practice it should take no longer than 10 minutes to put together this salad.

10+10 in 10 Chop Salad

A. Ingredients (I choose at least 10 of the following vegetables – choose your own 10 favorite vegetables to build your salad)

- Green lettuce: 2 kinds equivalent to 1 head (Romaine, green-leafy or red-leafy, oak-leaf, bib or butter – not iceberg)

- Spinach: couple of handfuls

- Sprouts: alfalfa, mung bean, clover, and/or mixed 3-bean

- Red vegetables: ½ cup tomatoes, ½ cup red bell peppers, ¼ cup radishes, ¼ cup red onion

- Orange/yellow vegetables: ¼ cup shredded carrot, ¼ cup orange or yellow pepper, ¼ cup shredded yellow squash

- Green vegetables: ½ cup cucumbers, ¼ cup green cabbage, 2 tbl. broccoli (chopped finely), ¼ cup snap peas, ¼ cup zucchini, ¼ cup green pepper, 1 avocado

- Purple vegetable: ½ cup purple cabbage

- White vegetable: ¼ cup cauliflower (chopped finely), 2 tbl. white onion

- Other additions for variety: sliced raw, unsalted nuts or seeds, whole beans (like black, kidney, or garbanzo), whole grains (like brown rice or couscous)

B. The "Must Have" Tools

- Large salad spinner – 10¼" in diameter (Note: no holes in the bottom)

- Large cutting board – 20¾" x 15"

- Chef's knife (sharp) with 8" blade, wider at handle

- Boning knife (sharp) with straight, narrow 6" blade

- Peeler

- Large bowl

- Two oversized spoons or fork and spoon for tossing

C. Directions

1. Take all ingredients out of refrigerator and wash. If possible, wash the vegetables as soon as you get home from the grocery store, so they are all ready to go. Or you can pre-wash veggies for at least two salads, so you only have to do this every other day.

2. Using a large salad spinner, spin the lettuce and spinach until very dry.

3. Finely chop lettuce and spinach – it's easier to chew – on large enough cutting board and fill a bowl large enough to contain a salad that will fill you up. (It takes time to learn how much salad is right for you.)

4. Finely chop vegetables and place on top of large bed of lettuce and spinach.

5. Squeeze ½ a lemon or lime over salad, along with a couple of shakes of balsamic vinegar (or any vinegar of choice).

6. Mix salad very well, until the avocado coats the lettuce and vegetables. The salad will shrink down by about one-fourth.

D. Helpful Hints

- Again, wash all green-leafy vegetables ahead of time, so they're ready when you're ready to eat a salad.

- Spin lettuce and spinach as dry as possible – they store better – and store in air-tight container.

- Make enough salad for lunch and dinner at one time, so you don't have to haul the stuff out twice. As for food preparation, make as little work for yourself as possible and enjoy your extra time doing something you love to do.

- Store all vegetables in the same area or, even better, the same storage bag in your refrigerator, so they are very accessible.

- Chop green-leafy vegetables and other vegetables very finely to make vegetables you may not be as fond of (or even hate) more palatable and easier to chew and digest.

E. Dressing the Raw

And what about the salad dressing? Great question.

When you make the conscious effort to feed yourself correctly with a big vegetable salad, it seems a bit self-defeating to smother it with a dressing concocted from calorie-loaded oil (yes, even olive oil), and added salt, sugar, creamy stuff, cheesy stuff and chemicals.

Remember this about salad dressing: the fat you eat is the fat you wear, whether is comes from an olive, a seed, a fish, or a cow.

Scout out the commercial salad dressings made with water, no sugar, and the fewest added chemicals. Read the labels. The local grocery store in my small area now has several no-oil, water-based dressings that can add different flavors to salads to make them more palatable and interesting to our spoiled taste buds.

What do I personally put on my salads?

Over the years I've tried dozens of commercially-made salad dressings. I gradually transitioned from using an oil-based dressing to a no-oil, water-based dressing, and then to making my own "dressing" of sorts so I knew exactly what was in it.

Quite frankly, I not only got tired of wondering what little devils may have snuck into those bottles (labels don't always reveal all), but I also got tired of the cost of special dressings. The result: I started making my own dressings, at first with olive oil. After all, don't we all know that olive oil is good for us? NOT! We best do the research on our own to flush out, once and for all, that slick lie that has slipped under the radar. Olive oil is good for one thing only: more calories, more fat, and more distance between you and your pants.

After reading about the harmful effects of all processed oils, including olive oil, I started creating a salad dressing that I now love. It took me about a week or so to get used to it, but once I did I could no longer stomach the heaviness and greasiness of those slimy added oils that add more ugly fat to our fat. Who needs it or wants it?

Here's my very complicated (just kidding!) recipe for salad dressing. Give it a good go. Try it for at least a week and then decide whether or not you like it. It will help to find a type of vinegar you like.

10+10 in 10 Salad Dressing

A. Ingredients

- 1 fill-you-up green-leafy salad with 10 different vegetables

- ½ of a fresh lemon or lime

- Organic balsamic vinegar (or any favorite vinegar)

(Bonus: almost no calories in dressing and extra nutrients from the lemon or lime)

B. Directions

- Step one: Cut one lemon or lime in half and use fingers to squeeze the juice out of the lemon or lime onto the salad.

- Step two: Give the bottle of balsamic vinegar a few shakes over the salad for desired amount.

- Step three: Mix very well. If an avocado has been added to the salad, the avocado coats the salad, giving it a wonderful flavor and texture, along with extra nutrients, without the disadvantages of a processed oil, including olive oil (see the fat section in Chapter 11).

When You Get Hungry, Eat!

After eating a large salad for lunch, you may get hungry in a couple of hours. Raw vegetables digest quickly. That's what's supposed to happen—good food goes in, moves through your stomach relatively quickly, and you get hungry again. It's a very simple and normal process.

This may come as a shock to you, but when you get hungry – eat! Whether it's an hour or three hours after your initial salad, snack on fresh, whole fruits; raw veggies, like cut-up or baby carrots, celery, cherry or grape tomatoes, cut-up cucumbers; raw, unsalted nuts, like almonds and pecans; and raw, unsalted sunflower and pumpkin seeds.

Is There Food after Salad?

Have no fear – you don't "have to" live on fruits and salads alone. Whew! What a relief!

For lunch, fill up on salad first with 10 different vegetables, about 80% of the time. If you want to eat something else after the salad, choose to take a break from salad altogether, or salad is not available, then go ahead and make other choices. Here are some alternatives to salad that are better for you than the typical American lunch.

1. A veggie sandwich with sprouted-grain bread such as Silver Hills or Ezekiel. Sprouted-grain bread is made from the sprouts of the wheat plant, rather than from the flour made from the ground-up wheat berries from the plant. The gluten in ground wheat berries is a fairly common allergen for many people. However, 100% whole wheat or whole grain bread is the best second choice after sprouted-grain bread.

   Here's a tidbit about whole wheat or whole grain bread, as we briefly discussed in Chapter 4. Just because bread is brown, doesn't mean it is whole grain. Breads consisting of mostly refined flours are often artificially colored. Always read the ingredients. For our purposes, bread is considered whole grain if it satisfies one or both of the following requirements: (1) Whole wheat flour is the only flour ingredient listed ("wheat flour" means white flour, *whole* wheat flour means whole wheat flour). (2) A whole grain (not wheat flour) is listed as the first ingredient, and the bread has a minimum of two grams of fiber per serving.

   Also, when I refer to whole grains in the 10+10 program, I am referring to true whole grains, as in brown rice, whole barley, or whole oats. Breads of any kind are not "whole grains." Rather, they are the final product of fragmented, ground, and highly processed grains. Breads are *not* your friends when it comes to maximum, steady weight loss, even if they are 100% sprouted or 100% whole grain. They are very dense and have hidden salt, oil, refined sugar, artificial coloring, flavoring, and preservatives. That's why breads, including those you make at home, are reserved for wiggling only! Even if homemade breads are made with 100% whole wheat, which most are not, they are made from highly processed flours, some kind of sweetener to feed the yeast, oil heated in the baking process (making cancer-causing free radicals), and salt. This combination of ingredients is not weight-loss or health friendly.

After you pick your bread, just as in the salad, pick your vegetables. Some of my suggestions are avocado, lettuce – the greener the better, spinach, tomato, cucumber, sprouts, bell pepper, onion, and shredded carrots. Then, you can add an optional spread, like mashed avocado, hummus, tahini, or a soy-mayonnaise substitute, such as Nayonaise, with only ten calories per tablespoon, and some unsweetened mustards.

2. A veggie wrap made with a whole wheat tortilla shell and your choice of the above vegetables or any vegetables of your choice.

3. A veggie sandwich made with whole wheat pocket pita bread.

4. A meatless, dairy-less, low-salt vegetable and/or bean soup.

5. A whole grain, such as brown rice or couscous, mixed with vegetables, as a cold or hot dish.

Or you may want a traditional sandwich with 100% whole wheat or sprouted-grain bread and the inner makings of your choice. Remember to ask yourself if that sandwich feeds you or depletes, and then make your decision. If you decide to eat it, should you feel guilty? Absolutely not! That's what wiggle room is all about – guilt-free eating of your favorites, 20% of the time. Then, be reasonable by returning to the "feed-me" foods the next meal or the next day.

WHAT "BIG BUTS" BLOCK YOUR WAY?

Okay, I said I'd get to them, and I know you probably have a lot. Go ahead and hit me with your best "big but shots" – I'm listening. I hope you'll listen back.

"But, but, but...salads don't fill me up."

I agree that the salads we are accustomed to eating, typically miniscule dinner salads or even medium-size lunch salads, will not fill you up. They certainly don't fill me up. When I eat in a restaurant, I often order double salads, and they still don't fill me up!

However, don't you think you could get full on a green-leafy salad with 10 different vegetables that is large enough to fill up the largest mixing bowl you have? Keep your mind open and give it a try. I promise you can make a salad large enough to fill you up. It will just take a lot more than you are used to.

"But, but, but...salads don't stick with me."

You are right again. Salads don't stick with you. Food goes in, food goes out. That's the normal course of digestion. Foods that feed you, not deplete you don't sit in your stomach like a big, ole' lump for hours on end. What's the solution to getting hungry again after filling up on salad? Eat – whether it's a half hour or two hours later.

Remember this. The meal you are eating is not your last meal (hopefully). You don't have to stuff yourself for fear of not getting food for a long, long time. This is America, and you can eat essentially any time, any place, anything you want.

And what if it's not convenient to eat again? Be sure you are fortified with quick, healthy easy-to-sneak snacks at all times. If circumstances won't allow you to eat exactly at the moment you'd like to eat, just wait a bit. You will not starve.

"But, but, but...I hate making salads."

I'll be the first to admit – I hate spending my time messing around with food. That's why I don't get the fuss about salads taking so much time to make. Goodness me. All you have to do is wash, chop, mix, and chew. You don't have to cook, measure, marinate, wait for the grill to heat, or use a blender. The only thing easier is a whole fruit.

But, for the sake of argument, I decided to find out exactly how long it takes me to make a salad. If I have pre-washed and stored the greens, it takes me no longer than 10 minutes, from start to finish, to make a salad – and that's one of my huge salads.

I think we women complain about making salads because we are used to making salads on top of preparing all the other foods for a meal. Yes, I agree. That's a pain, but not because of the salad preparation per se, but because of how complicated and time-consuming we make the entire meal.

A simple lunch with a 10+10 salad is mindless and the quickest way to get into your pants.

"But, but, but...it takes too much time to eat salad."

Yes, some of us actually moan and groan about how long it takes to eat a salad. As I've said before, 10+10 is going to require some moderate changes to your lifestyle. This is one of them. If you spend your time talking and eating lunch in a breakroom at work, you may have to spend a little more time chewing, and a little less time talking. But if the time it takes to chew and chew and chew bugs you, recall the mantra and say it in time to the rhythm of your chews: eating doesn't take time, it gives you time – when it counts – at the end of your life.

"But, but, but...it's a pain to bring salads to work, and I don't have a fridge to store them."

Again, I agree. I too hate to make a salad the night before or get up earlier to make one to bring to work. But the weight loss and health benefits are so worth the tiny bit of extra effort. And, if you have no refrigerator at work, do what I do – bring your salad in plastic bags in a little, hand-carried cooler. You can make as many excuses as you want. The bottom line is going to come down to your commitment to your body – your weight and your health. When there's a will, there's a way to get into those pants!

"But, but, but...I miss bread at lunch."

I can feel your pain – I love bread, too. I have a simple and not-so-brilliant solution.

To get your bread fix, how about eating a slice of sprouted-grain bread or 100% whole wheat bread after you fill up on that salad. Does that make you happier? You can eat it plain as lots of my clients do, or you can even throw some avocado and other vegetables on it.

Nix the butter, margarine, or regular mayonnaise most of the time – it's not worth the extra calories and fat that make direct beelines to your hips, thighs, stomach, breasts, arms, and butt, and pull you farther away from those pants. Remember: Big salad first, then a slice of bread, if that's your thing.

"But, but, but...I want something hot for lunch."

Have at it. Eat your salad first, and then enjoy the warm fuzzies that hot vegetable, bean, or split pea soup may offer you. Just be wary of salt, meat, and dairy that often come with soup. Lots of great recipes contain no meat, no dairy, and a minimum of salt. Look at the ingredients in canned soups. They are often full of the bad guys that sabotage weight loss, especially fat and salt. Choose your soups wisely.

"But, but, but...I'm so sick of salads that I just can't eat another one."

That's exactly what many of my weight-loss clients say to me after several weeks of eating salads, salads, and more salads. That flight from salads lasts about two days, and then they're back schmoozing with salads again. Why? Because they actually miss them. More importantly, they miss the way salads make their bodies feel.

Besides that, once they become aware of which foods feed them, help them lose weight, and get them closer to those pants, it's impossible to ignore these foods for very long.

If you shed your big buts and shift your thinking and your choices, you too will experience the inevitable craving for those foods that feed you, not deplete you – 10+10 vegetable salads, as well as whole, fresh fruits.

THERE'S NO TURNING BACK — IT'S YOUR TURN!

By noon or so, you have hit 10+10 with at least 10 different vegetables and around 10 whole, fresh fruits. Aren't you the smarty pants? That's not only food power – it's pants power!

Now that you've gained the fresh, plant foods momentum, don't stop now. The body you want is still waiting, and so is the last part of your eating day – dinner. Just imagine that electrifying feeling of putting both legs into those pants, gliding them over your hips, zipping the zipper, and buttoning that button easily. Those pants belong to YOU.

WHAT YOU NOW KNOW...

- Your beloved sandwich usually depletes you.
- For lunch, think raw, green, color, and quantity: a large, 10-veggie salad with oil-free, dairy-free salad dressing.
- Which big lunch buts keep you out of your pants.

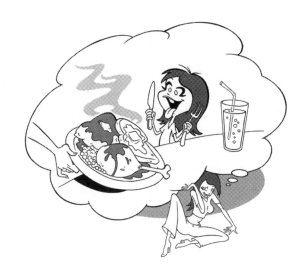

Chapter 8

Dinner: Shifting to Those Pants

What's up for dinner?

- What are your evening faves?

- What should you add for your 10+10 dinner?

- What "Big Buts" block your way?

"SUPPER'S READY. TIME TO EAT! "

Even though I haven't heard them spoken for over thirty-seven years, these five little words evoke memories, core-deep emotions, and even auto-salivary responses beyond my control. I can still smell the aroma of the different suppertime foods wafting up to my bedroom, tantalizing my appetite. I can still hear my mother's call, immediately followed by the predictable stampede of twelve little feet, scampering from our respective corners, filling the kitchen with chatter. I can still see all of us sitting at the table, in our pre-designated places with my father at the head, eight pairs of hands immediately diving into the food. My mouth still waters at just the thought of my favorite meal – baked chicken, mashed potatoes, and gravy. My mother knew – she saved the crispy, paprika wings especially for me.

It was my favorite meal of the day. And I wouldn't be surprised if it was yours, too. Probably still is.

Our memories keep us hooked forever into the dinners we grew up loving. We take enormous gratification in that final meal – it's like our reward for making it to the end of a day, for getting through work, school, or play. Dinnertime represents family time that can stir excitement or smooth the day's edges, reconnecting us to those we love and with whom we feel safe. Chicken, mashed potatoes, and gravy embody security, comfort, and love. To me, it embodies Mom.

So, is there any wonder why shifting our dinner habits is by far the most challenging food shift of all? As you start shifting the first two 10+10 meals of the day, fresh fruit for breakfast and a 10-veggie salad for lunch, the 10+10 way of eating becomes more and more appealing. With time and patience, it can even become effortless. However, it is much tougher to detach yourself from your oldest best friends at evening meals, despite their considerable contribution to calories, fat, and accumulated pounds – often more than the rest of the day. The unfortunate result: dinner can easily sabotage your earlier-in-the-day efforts to live (and lose) the 10+10 way.

WHAT ARE YOUR EVENING FAVES?

Let's talk about some of those all-American dinner darlings that possess the power to mesmerize, magnetize, and make your saliva flow. Besides baked chicken, mashed potatoes, and gravy (oh, yes!), there's also fried chicken, broiled chicken, barbequed chicken, and stewed chicken. Then there's roast beef, pot roast, chuck roast, steaks, hamburgers, and that mmm-mmm good comfort food, meatloaf.

To further titillate your demanding taste buds, you can always alternate the beef and chicken delights with turkey, pork, lamb, or seafood. For a bit of a change-up, how about some pasta smothered with tomato, meat, or cream sauce? Or you can combine the meat and pasta in dishes like beef stroganoff, chicken Alfredo, and tuna noodle casserole. And, of course, what would life have been like without mouth-melting macaroni and cheese?

But let's get real. You've come a long way from the days when mom made you dinner. While home-cooked traditional foods may still be your favorites, Americans don't eat just "American food" anymore. Nor, for that matter, do we eat food prepared at home as often. We've adopted fattier, meatier, cheesier, sweeter, and larger versions of ethnic favorites, such as Mexican burritos, Chinese takeout, Italian-style pizza, and Thai stir-fry. And we won't even get into that other choice: fast food.

Does Dinner Feed or Deplete Me?

Just like breakfast and lunch, take a close look at the typical foods you eat for dinner and ask yourself that all important 10+10 question: "Does this food feed me or deplete me?"

Sorry to say, none of the main dishes listed among your food faves in the previous section feed you. They all deplete, with the possible exception of mashed potatoes, if they come without butter, salt, or milk, so what's the point?

Of course, an ear of corn, a few spears of asparagus, and/or a small salad with iceberg lettuce, tomato, and cucumber drenched with oily salad dressing may tag along sometimes, but they're mere afterthoughts. We only care about the "star" of the meal, invariably meat, pasta, or another high-calorie, low-nutrient, ultra-filling main dish. Not exactly the right choices if you want to get into those pants!

Oh, dear. Now that all your dinner faves are suddenly blacklisted, along with the other deplete-me discards, you've got only one blaring question: "What's left to eat?" Don't panic – there's lots to eat that will fill you up and satisfy you, and you've got that wiggle room (if you must!) to visit your old dinner pals.

WHAT SHOULD YOU ADD FOR YOUR 10+10 DINNER?

Dinner is much simpler than you think. Just as you did for breakfast and lunch, you'll follow the 10+10 rules and fill up on the best-for-you foods first. **ADD** a salad to start with. Follow that with cooked vegetables, then grains and beans. **STOP** when you're full. **WIGGLE**, if you must, by eating some of your faves. Over time, you'll shift the best-for-you foods to the center of your meal, while your typical favorites transition to the sidelines.

Dinner can consist of up to four courses, eaten in order from the most nutrient-dense, low-calorie foods, to the lower-nutrient, higher-calorie foods. This way, you'll fill up on the good stuff. The courses will always go in this order:

First, add the 10-veggie salad, certainly the most nutrition for your calorie buck. As a time-saver, I often make enough salad at lunch to have a medium-sized serving left for dinner. Your dinner salad probably won't be as large as your lunch salad because of the other dinner foods you may choose to eat. However, make sure you eat enough to start filling your stomach. Some nights, you may eat a just large salad until you're full, and then stop. That would be an excellent dinner. But if you want more than a salad, move on to the next course.

Second, after you've eaten your salad, eat cooked vegetables. Select vegetables such as broccoli, cauliflower, green or yellow beans, spinach, peas, beets, or any one of your favorites. Prepare them however you like, as long as there's no added oil, butter, margarine, cheese, salt, sugar, or anything else from the deplete-me list. Steam them, sauté them in water, broil 'em, or throw them on the grill. And, by all means, add fresh herbs and spices for extra flavor.

If you're still hungry, be sure to prepare a denser vegetable, such as white potatoes (yes…free at last to eat white potatoes!), sweet potatoes, yams, or winter squash, like acorn or butternut. These vegetables are very filling – I promise! The easiest way to prepare them is to scrub or peel it, dice it, and throw it in a steamer. In literally 10 minutes, you can put the cooked potato or squash on a plate, mash it with a fork, and top it with any of these options:

- Pureed mixture of 1 avocado, 1 tomato, ¼ cup onions, ½ fresh lemon or lime, and herbs of choice

- Sautéed (in water) mushrooms, tomato, onions, and herbs and spices

- Fresh, grated garlic

- Fresh herbs and spices

- Fresh, chopped tomatoes

- Fresh, homemade salsa without salt

- Homemade tomato sauce without oil

Cooked vegetables help fill you up with the best-for-you foods while satisfying that "hot food" fix many of us crave at dinnertime.

Eating vegetables is like eating air – they offer very few calories for the nutrients. The more you add and fill up on salad and vegetables, the more quickly you'll get into those pants.

Third, if you're still hungry after you've eaten salad and cooked vegetables, add a whole grain and/or a whole legume (bean) dish as a change-up. These are also very filling. The options here are limited only by your imagination. Here's a small list of suggestions to get you started:

- Legumes (beans), either soaked overnight and cooked, or from a can without additives, preservatives, fat, or salt. These legumes can be kidney, black, pinto, or garbanzo beans or lentils and split peas. A great compliment to brown rice, and you can also throw these beans into your salads for a little added bulk.

- Whole grains. Try some brown rice, quinoa (pronounced keen-wah), whole wheat couscous, barley, buckwheat, millet, kasha, or whatever other whole grains they offer at your local grocer or farmer's market. Some of the grains (like the couscous) only take a few minutes to cook. Brown rice can take almost an hour. However, a relatively inexpensive rice cooker makes preparing whole grains a snap. Just wash the brown rice, put in rice cooker and cover with water, put the lid on, flip the "on" switch and in forty-five minutes or so, it's all done. You can put the same topping on these dishes as the ones for the potato, yam, or winter squash.

- Homemade polenta: mix 3/4 cup cornmeal into 2 cups boiling water, reduce heat, and stir until as thick as oatmeal. Mix or top with veggies.

- Meatless bean chili.

- Meat-free, non-dairy, low-salt, preferably homemade, vegetable and/or bean soups.

- Vegetable and bean tacos or burritos with whole wheat or corn tortilla shells, homemade guacamole, salsa, fresh tomatoes, onions, cilantro, herbs of choice, but, please, no cheese or sour cream.

- Occasionally, whole grain pastas with meat-free, non-dairy, non-oil, very low salt sauces. Pasta of any kind is highly refined so don't overdo it.

After three courses of plant foods, you should be full. If not, eat more until you're full. Then, if you really want to get into those pants, STOP.

Fourth, if you still want more food after eating all the plant foods, use your wiggle room. Choose the traditional meat, fish, or pasta you already made for you and your family. You'll automatically eat a much smaller portion because you're already full of the feed-me foods. How perfect is that? No deprivation. No war-of-the-wills. You simply can't eat any more. What a simple, effortless way of shaving off calories and pounds!

Remember – wiggle with caution. Be sure to keep your daily deplete-me foods under their 20 percent allowance. The fewer deplete-me foods you eat, the sooner you will get into your pants.

Dinner Recipes

Excellent choices for dinner abound, along with countless recipe books brimming with ideas and instructions. To expand your repertoire of whole plant food options, see the list of references at the end of this book. However, before you go recipe hunting, I strongly urge you first to master the basics of 10+10 for Life®. Concentrate on truly filling up first on raw and cooked vegetables, as well as their fresh fruit counterparts, and then venture into more time-consuming and complicated recipes if you choose. At first it's challenging enough to start shifting your thinking and food choices without making meals more complicated besides. It's too easy to get overwhelmed, discouraged, and just give up. And giving up is not an option! You have to live with yourself for the rest of your life.

After-dinner Munchies

What's it about after dinner that makes us want to eat? Do we get bored, restless, or just eat out of habit? Whatever the reason, eating too close to bedtime (less than two hours) interferes with burning calories efficiently during sleep. If we don't burn calories efficiently, then more fat gets stored in our fat – just what we don't want.

To combat this problem, I suggest that you "close the gate before the munchies get out of the barn." You know yourself well enough to anticipate whether you'll want to eat before bedtime. If you think you'll want a snack, eat it before it gets too close to bedtime. After all the effort you put into your day of eating the 10+10 way, for goodness sakes, make a healthy choice. Fresh fruit is a great evening snack, especially if you didn't get your full 10 fruits into the morning. If you aren't in the mood for fruit, eat some cut up veggies or some raw, unsalted seeds or nuts.

If you often get the munchies right before you go to bed, try breaking your habit by drinking a glass of water and just going to sleep. It'll be tough for a few weeks. But, when you wake up each morning, you'll be proud of yourself. And it will get easier.

WHAT "BIG BUTS" BLOCK YOUR WAY?

Oh, yes, just as with breakfast and lunch, I'm sure a few big buts threaten to block you from those pants. Let's beat a few of them back, one by one.

"But, but, but...I don't want to prepare more than one dinner, and my family likes the way we eat."

Just because you're transitioning your eating habits doesn't mean that your whole family has to change, unless you make that decision for them as their mom, aka dictator. Regardless of how your family eats, there's absolutely no need to prepare more than one dinner for you and your family. That's too much of a pain.

The best way to solve this problem is to prepare everything at once, as you would a normal dinner. Serve the salad, cooked vegetables, and a more filling dish, such as brown rice, along with the main entrée you've prepared for your family (and possibly for your fourth course). Just remember to eat in the 10+10 order, filling up on salad first, second on cooked vegetables, third, on denser foods like whole grains and/or beans, and, lastly, the traditional entrée or a small dessert. See? You and your family can be happy with one meal.

"But, but, but...my husband insists on eating meat every night."

Again, it doesn't matter whether or not your husband insists on eating meat. Just make one meal. Then he can eat the meat, and you can pick and choose what you want to eat out of the exact same meal. Meantime, your husband is as happy as a clam because you haven't tried to change his eating habits just because you have the urge to change yours – for the 100th time.

One more thing – it's easy to blame your husband or other family members for your reluctance to make changes. The only person who holds you back is you. No matter what someone else in your household eats, that person doesn't hold you down, hog tie you, pry open your jaws, and force food down your throat. You are responsible for you.

"But, but, but...I don't know how to cook any interesting vegetable dishes."

The beauty of vegetables is that they can be prepared quickly and simply – wash, chop, and chew. Raw is best and easiest. If you cook them, then wash, chop, steam, and chew. You can buy a no-fuss steamer for forty bucks that will last years and steam everything from vegetables to grains to meats, without fear of burning, scorching, or over cooking.

It's worth mentioning that the more you grow accustomed to the natural flavors of fruits and vegetables, the less inclined you will be to doctor them as prescribed in recipes. So-called interesting vegetable dishes make meal-planning, shopping, and preparing more time con-suming and complicated.

If you don't really enjoy cooking, stick with basics – especially at first. Then, if you get bored, get some vegan cookbooks or look at online recipes. Hundreds of resources for healthy vegetable dishes are available. Just make sure you choose recipes without unnecessary salt, sugar, oils, or animal products.

"But, but, but...I always crave sweets after dinner."

You could crave sweets for one of several reasons, or a combination thereof. For example, you could be addicted to refined sugar, as many Americans are. Or maybe you haven't eaten enough calories, and your body is telling you that you need to eat. Or perhaps you've gotten more than enough calories but not enough nutrients, and your body hunting for more nutrition.

Cravings often ease and even go away once you start feeding your body with nutrient-dense, energy-producing foods that satisfy your hunger drive, as in whole, fresh fruits and vegetables. When you get that urge for something sweet, eat fruit. Keep working at it. The longer you stay away from refined sugar, the easier it is to break out of that sugar trap, and those extra calories and layers.

"But, but, but...we entertain guests and eat out more than 20% of the time."

The bottom line is this: your social life is your choice, and what you eat while you socialize is also your choice. If you're really serious about getting into those pants, then you can choose to do one of two things: change your social life so you have more control over your eating environment, or change your eating habits while you socialize.

Here are a few suggestions when you're in a social whirlwind:

- When you're going to a friend's to eat, be honest and say you'd love to enjoy her company, but may you please bring a salad and vegetable so that you can continue your eating plan without creating extra work for her.

- Eat a large salad before you go out to eat so you aren't very hungry, and you'll naturally be happy eating less of the not-so-good for you food.

- When entertaining at home, make sure you include in your meal those 10+10 foods that you can fill up on first.

- Choose restaurants that you know serve at least some good-for-you foods.

- Remember, this is not your last meal. If you can't find enough feed-me foods to eat and you're doing so well with the 10+10 plan that you don't want to indulge in deplete-me foods, then just don't eat – or at least not much. It's not a big deal. This is America - there's plenty to eat when you get home.

"But, but, but…I don't have time to make dinners with several courses."

No doubt it takes time to learn which food-me foods work best for you and your family, shop for those foods, and then prepare them. But, it gets easier with practice and with simplification of meals.

Here are some hints to help streamline meal-making:

- Pre-prepare foods when you can. For instance, pre-wash fruits and vegetables when you get them home from the store. Also, wash and spin dry your lettuce and spinach for your salads a couple of days ahead of time and store in an air-tight container. Pre-chop your salads up to two meals ahead, but not more. That way everything is ready when you need it.

- When you make your lunch salad, while you have all the stuff out, make enough salad for dinner, too. Or, if you prefer, make your salads at dinnertime, take a dinner portion out, and leave most for lunch the next day. Salad can be made ahead, as long as you wait to dress it until you're ready to eat.

- If you are really crunched for time, you can buy pre-washed, prepackaged lettuce, spinach, baby carrots, and all kinds of vegetables in certain grocery stores, although it's best to wash and chop them yourself. Foods start losing nutrients and enzymes the minute you wash and cut them.

- Steam, rather than bake, potatoes, yams, and squash in much less time.

- Prepare brown rice in a rice cooker and bean dishes and soups ahead of time, such as on the weekend.

- Use the right kitchen tools to prepare your meals, such as a good salad spinner, a sharp chef knife, and a large cutting board. This will save time and help you avoid frustration.

- Organize your kitchen and refrigerator as efficiently as possible. I put all the vegetables I use for salads in one place, often in one large plastic bag. I keep the veggies on one side of the refrigerator, fruits on the other. The fruits and veggies that don't need refrigeration are well-organized in bowls on my countertop or in my pantry.

- Keep meals as simple as possible. Usually the simpler the meals are, the better they are for you. When you get down to it, you really don't have to make several courses for dinner at all, at least not for yourself. Make sure all your greens and vegetables are washed ahead of time, and in just 10 minutes you can whip up the most nutrient-packed, weight-reducing full course meal you can imagine – one big 10+10 salad with at least 10 different vegetables, flavored with lemon and balsamic vinegar!

I'll repeat this one more time: taking time to eat correctly doesn't take time it gives you time – when it counts – at the end of your life.

Most importantly of all, if you have the right mindset with clear intentions and a vision for yourself, you'll be happy to reprioritize and organize your life around your new food habits. Those very foods and habits will get you into those pants and keep you there!

10+10 Is Simple, Not Always Easy

So there you are – we've gotten through your 10+10 food day (we'll get to beverages in the next chapter). Look at how much you've already learned:

- ADD and fill up on foods that feed you – fresh, whole fruit for breakfast, a big 10+10 veggie salad for lunch, and good-for-you foods for dinner.

- STOP eating when you're satisfied and full.

- WIGGLE (if you must!)

You have to admit – that sounds simple enough, doesn't it? Well, it is simple. And the best part is – it works! The whole package can be yours: smaller pants size, how-does-she-do-it looks from other women (the kind you used to secretly give), a better sex life, a healthier outlook, fewer medications, and the works.

However, simple doesn't always translate into easy. Roadblocks always loom before us: spoiled taste buds, nay-sayers, those pesky big buts, and our own self-doubt. But with your bulldogged persistence, patience, and that vision of you prancing in those pants (way to go!), you can become the body you want to be.

WHAT YOU NOW KNOW...

- We all love our all-American, deplete-me dinners, centered on meat, fish, pasta, dairy products, and brown-colored white bread.

- To lose weight, eat dinner foods in this order:

    1. First, a veggie salad with a no-oil, no-dairy, no-chemical dressing.

    2. Next, steamed veggies of choice, like broccoli, cauliflower, green beans, asparagus.

    3. Followed by more filling veggies: potatoes, sweet potatoes, yams, winter squash (no butter, margarine, or sour cream please) or a whole grain, like brown rice.

    4. And, very last, if you must: traditional American foods, like beef, chicken, fish, or pasta.

- Which big dinner buts keep you out of your pants.

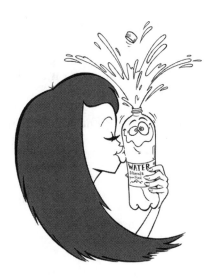

Chapter 9
Let's Drink to Your Pants

What's up for beverages?

- What do you drink now?

- What are better choices?

Now that you know how to slim down with 10+10 foods, let's make sure you don't drown your new healthy, slimmer self in your drinks.

WHAT DO YOU DRINK NOW?

What do you drink in a typical day? Give it some thought. If you're like most Americans, you get almost one quarter of your daily calories from beverages. In fact, the single largest calorie contributors to the American diet are sodas and other sweet drinks.

Most fad diets and eating plans don't even deal with beverages. But, they are so important! After all, you drink nearly every time you eat, and in between meals, too. What you drink has a huge impact on your caloric intake, as well as the amount of nutrients you get, or don't get, in a day.

So, what do you drink? Let's start with your morning. Are you a water kind of gal? Do you drink freshly squeezed orange juice? Coffee or tea? Milk? Diet shakes? Protein drinks?

How about lunch and dinner? Maybe it's more coffee, or just water. Perhaps you break into the sodas or sports drinks. Maybe it's another diet shake. Or, maybe you're into fruit juices.

Whatever your drinking preferences, it's important to do the same feed-me/deplete-me analysis you did for breakfast, lunch, and dinner. Think about all the drinks you consume in a typical day and ask yourself the question: "Which drinks feed and which ones deplete?"

Keep in mind, it's not just about calories. Go back and look at the feeding/depleting chart in Chapter 5 one more time. The caffeine, alcohol, sugars, artificial sweeteners, chemicals, dyes, preservatives and/or salts in most drinks are extremely depleting. Drinking depleting drinks, just like eating depleting foods, interferes with both weight loss and health gain.

As the chart in Chapter 5 shows, the only beverages that don't deplete are water, caffeine-free herbal teas, fresh, homemade fruit and vegetable juices, and raw, unpasteurized, store-bought juices (a rare breed).

All other drinks deplete to some degree, even the 100% commercial fruit and vegetable juices. Surprised? Let's go through some of your deplete-me favorites one by one.

Coffee and Caffeinated Tea

Brace yourself for this one – it may hurt a bit. I can understand why coffee, along with caffeinated tea, could seem like the ideal beverage when you're trying to lose weight. After all, it has zero calories, **if** you drink it black and don't add the extra calories from sugar, chemical sweeteners, cream, or milk. However, those zero calories hardly compensate for the fact that coffee depletes you – big-time. More than just calories can sabotage your weight and health.

No two ways about it, coffee contains many of these other body-unfriendly things, not the least of which is everyone's favorite drug, caffeine. Caffeine is an addictive stimulant. Even decaffeinated coffee contains caffeine, though in smaller amounts. We drink coffee to get that addictive wake-up buzz. And if you don't believe you're hooked, try weaning yourself off it, and see what happens. A killer headache for days – a sure sign you're addicted.

Aside from being addictive, coffee is associated with depression, diarrhea, atherosclerosis (hardened arteries), rheumatoid arthritis, urinary incontinence, reduced insulin sensitivity, and the leaching of calcium from bones, osteoporosis. It is a natural diuretic, overworking your kidneys and bladder. If your organs work harder, guess what happens? You wear down faster – that's called aging!

As for that quick pick-me-up you want, caffeine may seem to give you energy with its deceptive, artificially-stimulated highs, but those highs are always followed by bottom-out lows. These spikes and dips drain your natural resources for sustainable energy.

Soda

You might as well take some of your household chemicals, add some sugar, and drink up. After all, some sodas, like Coke, can remove rust from a car's engine.

If that isn't creepy enough, how about the fact that most 12 oz. cans of pop contain about ten teaspoons of sugar, not to mention the super-sized, fast-food sodas as big as 42 ounces? This represents a significant portion of the 33 teaspoons of sugar the average American eats a day, amounting to over ten pounds a month or about twenty percent of daily calories. We're trying to get weight off, not drink more on! Both regular and diet soda are statistically linked to obesity, tooth decay, caffeine dependence, type 2 diabetes, and weakened bones. Further, the aspartame in diet sodas is believed to be toxic to the body.

Also, drinking soda tends to increase cravings for other sweets, leading to uncontrollable bingeing. It's ultra-depleting, addictive, and laden with chemicals, sugar, and calories that hinder your weight loss.

In a word, yuck! Why would you put something like that into your body at all, much less multiple times a day? Switch to sparkling water if you need the fizz. Anything but soda.

Protein Drinks

Protein drinks are chemical concoctions with added sugar, salt, and calories. Plus, they overload you with protein when you're probably already getting too much (a fact which will be discussed in detail in Chapter 11). But, for purposes of this chapter, it's sufficient to say that if you're trying to lose weight, there's no reason to drink chalky, powdery, high-calorie protein drinks. Make a fresh fruit smoothie instead. It tastes much better, provides great nutrition with plenty of protein (yes, fruit contains protein), and contains no chemicals or additives.

Processed Juices

Unless store-bought fruit and vegetable juices are marketed as raw and fresh, they are cooked and processed, wiping out all enzymes and many vitamins. Basically, all you're getting is cooked, concentrated fruit sugar, usually with added chemicals and preservatives.

Furthermore, many fruit juices contain additional refined sugars, unless they specifically say "unsweetened." Believe it or not, even those that say "no sugar added" may have added some form of refined sugar. Processed vegetable juices fare no better. They're usually loaded with salt, sugar, and questionable manmade chemicals for flavoring and preserving.

Regardless of what has been added to processed juices, they offer you too many calories for too few nutrients. Read the label before you drink. If a juice contains added sugars, salt, preservatives, colorants, or if it's pasteurized, it falls into your 20% wiggle room category.

Alcohol

At this point in your life, you know that alcohol is good for two things – getting tipsy and adding calories. Two glasses of red wine, for example, contain about as many calories as a large salad, an entire 10+10 lunch. Cutting out alcohol is an easy way to cut down calories.

People make endless excuses for drinking alcohol. No more excuses. Alcohol is a drug, a depressant. It depletes, and it's addictive. Rationalizing that alcohol is derived from "good-for-you" plants, like wine from red grapes or beer from wheat, is like saying you get the daily vegetables you need from the mustard, ketchup, pickles, and potato chips you eat with your burger.

If you drink alcohol, you drink for one reason – because you want to. Period.

WHAT ARE BETTER CHOICES?

Water

Now that I've berated your favorite drinks, let's talk about better choices. Of all the dozens of different drinks now commercially marketed, water is the best at its job: hydrating. And it comes with zero calories, zero chemicals, zero sugar, and zero salt, all for the price of zero dollars. Drinking water restores fluids in our bodies, which we lose constantly through elimination, breathing, and sweating.

I know – boring. No, boring is being straight-jacketed to a kidney dialysis machine three hours a day, three days a week because you didn't eat the right foods and drink the right drinks. Now, back to the not-so-boring water.

Interestingly enough, water neither feeds nor depletes. It's neutral, but critical for a well-functioning body. The same goes for herbal teas that say "naturally caffeine-free," list only plants as ingredients, and contain no manmade chemicals.

But I Don't Like the Taste.

The taste? I just don't get that. Water is tasteless, or should be if it's pure and clean. The ideal beverage isn't meant to schmooze your bratty taste buds. It's supposed to keep you adequately hydrated and alive. Besides that, your tastes are probably so whacked out from eating over-sugared, over-salted, over-flavored foods and drinks for so long that you might not even have a true sense of what tastes good anymore. When you start 10+10, your tastes will change dramatically.

Try sticking to water for a month while you give 10+10 a try. If you need a change up from water, try flavoring it with freshly squeezed lemon, lime, or orange juice or drink caffeine-free herbal tea. Then reassess your tastes to see whether it's really as bad as you thought, or whether your taste buds had just been tainted by sensory overload.

Bottled or Tap?

I will sidestep that debate altogether here. Just make sure your water is clean and pure. If your tap water has high amounts of an element that is bad for you, buy a good filtration system, or buy bottled. Keep in mind, however, that bottled water is not regulated, so it's impossible to tell whether the bottled water you're buying is clean and pure.

How Much Water?

Believe it or not, I've incited more riots than I care to admit when answering this question because my answer is: I have absolutely no idea!

But luckily you do. You know exactly how much water you need at any given moment. You were gifted with an amazing instinct that keeps you fully hydrated *if* you listen to it. It's known in our language as thirst. When you are thirsty, drink (water!). When your thirst is quenched, stop drinking. When you're thirsty again, drink. It doesn't get much simpler than that.

Somewhere along the way, drinking eight glasses a day became a decree that we all believed. But the truth is, your water needs vary according to your size, the types of foods you eat, the climate, and your activity levels. So there's no magical amount.

For instance, if you load up on high-salt foods, like meat, cheese, processed foods, chips, and salty snacks, you will need to drink more water than if you fill up on fresh fruits and vegetables. Fresh fruits and vegetables contain a lot of water and little sodium, reducing your need for drinking water.

Most importantly, pay attention to your thirst cues, carry water with you, and drink whenever and however much your body tells you.

Freshly-made Juices

Juices, freshly made from whole, raw fruits and vegetables, are another great beverage choice. They not only hydrate perfectly like water, but they feed as well, providing essential vitamins, minerals, phytochemicals, enzymes, and macronutrients. These liquid foods quench your thirst and offer top value for your calorie buck at the same time!

Your best option is to make your own fresh fruit and vegetable juices using an efficient juicer. If, like me, you're already making juices, then great. I've been juicing regularly for close to thirty years. But, if this is a new concept for you, you may want to wait until you're really comfortable with the 10+10 way of eating before adding one more thing to think about.

For now, do just one thing: Consider nixing all the beverages you drink except pure, clean water. If you want a hot drink, try some naturally caffeine-free herbal tea. Your pocketbook and hips will thank you.

Recap

You finally made it to the point in the book where you have all the basic knowledge you need to launch into 10+10! We've covered breakfast, lunch, dinner, snacks, and beverages. You also have a good handle on the concept of feeding vs. depleting, a valuable tool that will help you make better choices, starting today.

After being introduced to a brand new way of thinking about foods and beverages, I'm sure you have lots of questions and concerns.

That's a good thing – that means you're trying to process all that you've learned. And, don't worry, I'll get to many of your questions and Big Buts in the next few chapters. For now, be patient with yourself. Learning anything new takes time.

Congratulations to you for having the guts and conviction to shift your thinking, shift your choices, shift your habits, and shift your cute, littler behind right into those pants! Be ever so grateful and proud of all that you are right now, while you strive to evolve into all that you can be.

WHAT YOU NOW KNOW...

- Beverages contribute 25% of daily calories consumed, translating into extra fat that keeps you out of your pants.

- Most beverages deplete with sugar, sugar substitutes, protein, colorings, preservatives, chemicals, alcohol, and/or caffeine.

- Water is the best beverage for simple hydration.

- Drink when thirsty. The more fruits and vegetables you eat, the less water you need.

- Fresh, homemade fruit and vegetable juices, liquid feed-me food, both hydrate and feed you.

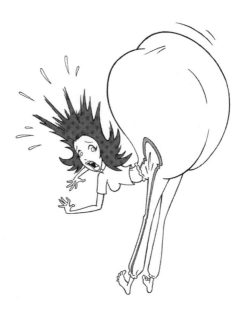

Chapter 10

21 'Big Buts' Between You and Your Pants

- Big Buts Stop You from Starting

- Big Buts Sabotage You Along the Way

- Food-Specific Big Buts

- Other People's Big Buts

ope. That's what your introduction to 10+10 and its revolutionary, yet simple weight-loss principles have given you. You allow yourself to let go of past experiences and dream of the possibilities. What if you really could get slim and fit, without starving, sacrificing, and depriving? What if you could feel better about your body and yourself? What if that one feat that has always eluded you – losing fat forever – could open up your world beyond imagination?

And then a pivotal moment occurs. That spark of hope ignites into a single, positive thought: "I can do it. This time, I'm going to get into those pants – no matter what!"

Even though you mean it, it's not long before your head floods with the daunting "to-do's." Planning, creating a new grocery list, shopping, shifting meal preparation, and breaking the news of your new routine to your family. It all boggles your brain, making you moan out loud.

Hope falters – stymied by your overwhelming self-doubt, calling forth the "yeah, buts" – that endless parade of excuses that threaten to thwart your good intentions one more time.

The invasion of the "yeah, buts" is predictable. But together, we can flush them out into the open, break them down into little pieces, chew them up, and spit them right back out, rendering them powerless to stop you from realizing your body-dream-come-true.

BIG BUTS THAT STOP YOU FROM STARTING

"Yeah, but...this way of eating is just too radical."

Change is tough. Change beyond what you can envision for yourself is perceived as radical, unreachable.

Our old ways of eating bring comfort. It is familiar, mindless, and soothing. By contrast, transitioning into wrapping your day around fresh fruits and vegetables and letting go of favorite foods is uncomfortable, disruptive, effortful – even radical. And, it's scary. You just can't take another disappointment in yourself for failing to do something you want so badly – to lose weight.

But sometimes, in order to reach a worthy goal, it takes nothing short of radical. Nothing else has worked. And what goal is more worthy than transforming the possibility into the reality of stepping into your body-dream-come-true?

Sure, it takes blood, sweat, and lots of tears to shake up your world of food and turn it inside out and upside down. But just think of the rewards – the opportunity for growth, the catalyst for self-evolvement, the adventure into the brand new and unknown, and the exhilaration of getting into those pants. Ah, those pants!

Like you said yourself, my friend, you can do this. It's your time. Keep that vision of yourself in your mind's eye at all times. Set your sails and follow your own true north, no matter how stormy it gets, no matter how radical it seems.

You not only can do it, you *will* do it!

"Yeah, but...I get no support."

It's uncomfortable to feel as though you're alone in your struggle. I've got to be brutally honest here. You will feel as though you're alone because, in fact, you are. Chances are no one else in your immediate world will think and eat like you. When you start listening to your own guts about your body and your life, it's very likely no one you know will hear that same voice. It's a lonely and scary place to be.

Your life partner, no matter how loving, may think, "Oh, no, here we go again." Your kids, no matter how grown up, may scoff, "You're crazy, Mom, and by the way, could you pleeeease make my favorite roast beef, gravy, and mashed potatoes with your great apple pie for dessert?" And your dear friends, no matter how much they "yes" you, may undermine your intentions with inappropriate gestures and comments like, "Please join me. Just one piece of chocolate won't matter – besides, haven't you heard, it's good for you (500 calories and all!)."

Your changing may be difficult, if not impossible for them to understand. It may be inconvenient. It could even be threatening. After all, your example may force them to think about their own food issues and habits, and they just may not be ready for that. Your timing to make changes may not be in sync with their agenda.

But, in spite of that lack of support from all sides, listen to that inner voice that pleads with you. No matter how lonely you get when creating your brand-new food day with the best-for-you foods, it's way more lonely to battle cancer, to get a leg cut off from diabetes, or to insulate yourself from making love to your husband because you're too embarrassed to show your body.

Yes, you do need support. We all do, but seek it elsewhere. Just put up your antenna and attract those few key people and resources that will feed your flame. It could be a website, a newsletter, a knowledgeable mentor, an author who resonates with you, or a new friend you meet at the organic produce section in the store.

When you get your own intentions crystal clear, you will attract all the people, support, and material assistance you need to help you on your solo and noble journey. And I hope you can feel me cheering the unique and beautiful you all along the way!

"Yeah, but...I already eat a healthy enough diet, and I'm still overweight."

Whether or not you think you eat "well enough," "balanced enough," "moderate enough," or "vegetarian enough," if you're still overweight, it's not enough. The evidence is pretty clear – you wear it. If you're serious about losing that weight, you must do more.

Of all the "yeah, buts," I find complacency, or self-satisfaction, the hardest one to break through. If you are this type of person, you "think," or even "know" that you eat "the right way," no matter what that way happens to be. There's no more room for improvement, even though your body tattles a different tale.

The bottom line is this: you can't be helped until you're open and ready to be helped. But, since you are this far along in the book, I'm guessing this is not you. You wouldn't be investing your energy and valuable time with me unless you were not only ready, but eager.

Don't be deceived by the old, worn-out measuring stick you're using – the infamous Four Food Groups. To most, moderation and balanced are perceived as eating enough, but not too much of each traditional food from the Four Food Groups – meat, cheese, cereal, bread, and a few fruits and vegetables thrown in. Contrary to popular belief, true balanced eating is filling up on only nature's best: fresh fruits and vegetables, along with whole grains, beans, raw nuts, and seeds, with no added oils, salt, sugar, or manmade chemicals. Then, the instant your brain says you're full, you stop eating

As for moderation, sadly, our collective excess fat clearly demonstrates that we Americans have no clue what moderation means.

Furthermore, the self-proclaimed, lofty "vegetarian" or "vegan" status too often licenses a diet of plant foods loaded with oil, salt, and sugar. After all, you can gorge yourself on French fries, tortilla chips, and chocolate and still be considered a "vegetarian," even though you eat lots of terribly unhealthy foods. The label you give yourself is not important. What you feed yourself is.

Look in the mirror. If you're unhappy with what you see, then you should not be satisfied with your food and lifestyle choices. Yes, be proud and happy with every one of your baby steps to better yourself, but always give yourself more wiggle room for opening the next door and stepping up to that next level of awareness and improvement to meet your body-best ideals for yourself.

"Yeah, but...I don't like to feel different."

The truth is, when it comes to weight loss and your health, you should allow no one to sabotage the decisions you know are right for you. You, and you alone, are the one who has to live and, ultimately, die with the decisions you've made. And it may mean being different from everyone around you.

When my lovely daughter, Erin (now in her late twenties) and I feel different from everyone else, and lonely because of it, we remind each other of one fundamental truth that I taught her years ago: you've got to *be* different to *make* a difference.

You may be different with respect to the food and lifestyle choices you make and uncomfortable at times because of it, but be proud and grateful that you have the knowledge, the awareness, and the bulldog persistence to swim against the whims and follies of our culture and not just survive, but thrive.

Your difference and quiet example speak volumes about your inner strength. They not only powerfully impact your life, but impact the lives of those around you. Feel your difference. Understand your difference. Live in accordance with your difference. And, above all else, appreciate your difference, a precious and rare gift. That very difference can give you life itself and lots of fun all along the way – especially getting into those pants!

BIG BUTS THAT SABOTAGE YOU ALONG THE WAY
"Yeah, but...a little bit won't kill me."

You're so right. A little bit of anything won't kill you.

No, one breakfast of eggs, bacon, white bread and butter will not kill you. Two cups of coffee a day will not kill you. One doughnut in the morning will not kill you. One piece of pizza (and who eats just one piece?) will not kill you. One ham and cheese on rye will not kill you. One dish of ice cream will not kill you. One glass of wine will not kill you. (I could go on for a very long time with this list.)

One of anything will not kill you. The problem is that these are the very foods that typically fill the stomachs of most Americans every day, all day. When you stack up these "ones" day after day, week after week, and year after year, these "ones" will very likely do just that – kill you.

"Yeah, but…I crave sweets, and when I go on a sugar binge, I can't stay away."

As you have been reminded over and over, refined sugars are addictive. Often you get pulled right back into that sugar trap after indulging in it – even just once.

Be aware of the sugar demon you're facing. When you fall victim, get back to 10+10 quickly. When you crave sugar, eat fruit, fruit, and some more fruit. It's a sweet alternative that is key to crushing those sugar cravings. And, believe it or not, vegetables help cut the cravings, too.

"Yeah, but…I will get bored eating like this."

Why is it that the same chocolate, coffee, ice cream, baked goodies, breakfast cereal, sandwich, pizza, hamburgers, fries, and diet pop never get boring when we eat them day after day? Our taste buds are spoiled by the sugared-up, salted-up, flavored-up, fattened-up foods and drinks we're conditioned to eat and love. Most Americans eat a surprisingly small variety of foods from day to day.

The sheer magnitude of vegetable and fruit varieties opens a world of possibilities. They come to us outfitted in a vast assortment of colors, shapes, sizes, textures, and tastes. If you give your taste buds a chance, they can change to accommodate a new array of the natural, undoctored flavors of whole, fresh plant foods. Be patient with yourself! You'll get there. After a while, delight and appreciation for nature's best will replace boredom.

"Yeah, but...there are temptations everywhere."

Goodness me. Tempting foods lurk everywhere you go – at home, work, the store, your friend's, Costco, the gym, the movies, the DVD store on every corner on every street in your all-American town... everywhere. What's a girl to do when she's trying her hardest to stay the course? Keep good-for-you foods with you at all times – at home, work, in the car, when visiting – and stay full on these foods. Temptations then magically drop away.

"Yeah, but...I love to eat in restaurants and don't want to give that up."

You can still eat in restaurants. But for the most part, include these meals as part of your wiggle room. Sometimes you can make some excellent choices while eating out, sometimes they are less than ideal. What I do is look at the menu and find out which plant foods are offered and choose from them. For instance, I will choose their best vegetable salad with the dressing – oil-free if possible – on the side and sometimes a double salad. I might also order a baked potato with steamed vegetables on the side and put the vegetables on the potato.

That's very filling. Also, many restaurants serve vegetable side dishes and will prepare a special dish if you tell them you don't eat meat or dairy. Like I said in Chapter 5, raw is better than cooked, plant is better than animal, and no oil is better than any oil.

"Yeah, but...I'm going on vacation for a month."

Have fun and don't worry about the food, especially if you are just starting out! A vacation is not an ideal time to make a lifestyle change because you are out of your normal routine. Make better choices when you can, but for the most part relax and go with the flow or you could drive yourself crazy. Just be sure you are right on track before you go. Then, as soon as you get back, get right back on 10+10.

"Yeah, but...what about all the G-A-S?"

No doubt about it. Fruits and vegetables, energy-charged, nutrient-dense, fiber-rich, low-calorie foods, come loaded with carbohydrates. And that smells, no, spells G-A-S, so sorry to say. Give a hearty welcome to your colon's frequent guest – one of the signs you're on the right track. That said, even though gas is normal, you may still want to avoid getting blown up like a helium-filled balloon.

When you first start eating 10+10, your intestines may go through a cleaning up and clearing out phase, and gas is the natural byproduct of this process. With time, gas production should decrease. Be patient.

Be aware of the few gas-pumping champs: legumes, fruits combined with other foods, and calciferous vegetables like broccoli, cauliflower, and cabbage. Chopping the vegetables very finely for salads, cooking them, and chewing well may help. Regarding legumes, you can try several gas-reducing hopefuls:

- Soak the beans overnight and throw out that water. Boil them in fresh water.

- Don't eat fruit, desserts, or any other sweet stuff with beans.

- Try a commercial digestive enzyme, like Bean-o. It works for some (though not for me).

- Eat smaller sized legumes, such as lentils and split peas, rather than larger beans like kidneys and pintos. Smaller beans are often easier to digest.

- Eat small quantities of beans. Avoid over eating them.

Fruits can increase fermentation of carbohydrates and rotting of meat in the colon. The result: gas. My advice is to eat fruit in the morning, without the addition of other foods, until about one hour before lunch, as I discussed in the breakfast chapter. In addition, do not eat fruit for dessert, with a meal or immediately after one. Wait two to three hours after a meal before eating fruit. Eat melons alone, without other foods (including fruits).

Lastly, exercise. That daily walk does way more than move your heart, lungs, muscles, joints, and blood; it moves the gas out, and in a hurry!

"Yeah, but...losing 2.5 pounds a month seems so slow."

I'm with you. I wish I could wave a magic wand over you, melt away the pounds, and give you a new body – instantly. But, unfortunately, neither one of us will get our wish that fast. However, the wish can come true – it just takes time and patience.

Yes, losing 2.5 pounds a month, the weight loss goal I often recommend in 10+10, may initially seem painfully slow, but those bite-size 2.5 pounds set you up for success, not for failure. Look at it this way. If you attain that very doable goal of losing 2.5 pounds every month for twelve months, that adds up to the grand total of thirty pounds! We all know how fast a year goes by. How would you feel if you were thirty pounds lighter this exact time next year? Pretty good, don't you think?

And the best part – it doesn't end there. You can continue to transition to eating better and better over the long haul. In another twelve months, you could be down another thirty pounds, for the even grander total of sixty pounds! Whoa! Wouldn't you be beyond thrilled with yourself and deserve to be! And all it took was 2.5 pounds a month – slow and steady as she goes.

FOOD-SPECIFIC BIG BUTS

"Yeah, but...I don't like _____." (Fill in the blank with your most hated plant-based food.)

Okay. So you don't like broccoli or cauliflower or spinach or brown rice or apples or kidney beans or whatever. Two points here.

First, hundreds of fruits, vegetables, whole grains and beans vie for your attention. Explore your local grocery store or go to Wikipedia. com for an extensive list. If you don't like something, choose something else. It's that simple.

Second, if you think you dislike all vegetables, introduce them one at a time, little by little. For instance, if you don't like a particular vegetable that could go into your 10+10 salad, chop it very finely. You'll find that when a vegetable is cut up so finely that you can hardly see it, you can hardly taste it either. Introduce disliked vegetables one at a time this way. And what if you still don't like them? I say, who cares?

Eat them anyway – your life depends on it, and that should be enough reason to eat them. Hold your nose if you have to. I used to think avocados were disgusting. Now I love them and eat at least two a day. Your tastes will change with time – I promise.

"Yeah, but...I love my _____."
(Fill in the blank with your favorite deplete-me food.)

Oh, dear. Do I sense a bit of whining here? Of course you love cheese/meat/sandwiches/chocolate/cola/potato chips/whipped cream. We all do.

But just because you love something doesn't mean you have to eat it, especially not all the time! To reach your weight and health goals, you have to change the way you *think* about food. That doesn't mean you will change how you feel about your food favorites. It just means when you follow the 10+10 rules and fill up on the best-for-you foods first, many of your food faves slip out of your life, almost without your noticing – especially after you start seeing results. Does that mean you love those faves any less? Not at all. I haven't had a chicken, mashed potatoes, and gravy dinner for close to twenty years, and I still swoon just with the thought of it!

Additionally, don't forget the third 10+10 rule: wiggle (if you must)! 10+10 is **not** about having to give up anything. It's about getting to add the foods that feed you, not deplete you. If you want some cheese/meat/caviar/spam once in a while, have at it – just remember not to wiggle more than 20% of the time.

"Yeah, but...if I don't eat enough meat, where do I get my protein?"

By far, this question is the very first most people ask me when they first learn about 10+10. Hang on a bit longer – it will be answered in Chapter 11. This question is so important that it deserves a chapter of its own.

"Yeah, but...if I don't have dairy, where do I get my calcium?"

This is the second most common question people ask me. It will be addressed in Chapter 14.

"Yeah, but...what about vitamin B12?"

Plant foods are rich with vitamins, with the exception of vitamin B12, which is produced by tiny microorganisms in the intestines of animals and in the soils. When plant foods are grown in rich soils, they can absorb vitamin B12. However, if plants are grown in depleted soils, they may not contain this vitamin. Furthermore, our cleaning practices wash away all remnants of vitamin B12 right along with the soil.

Luckily, the body stores this B12 for about three years. Taking small amounts of vitamin B12 in supplement form will assure you of getting all you need. You can also get the levels in your blood checked if you question it.

"Yeah, but...how do I get iron?"

Contrary to popular belief, eating a variety of plant foods typically provides more iron than meat does. Not only that, certain products, like dairy products, coffee, and eggs inhibit the absorption of iron. On the other hand, many fruits and vegetables are rich in iron (e.g. dark green vegetables, mushrooms, nuts, seeds), and several others are rich in vitamin C, which helps improve the absorption of iron (e.g. bell peppers, snow peas, broccoli, cauliflower, cantaloupe, oranges, grapefruits, and strawberries, to name a few).

To give you an idea of comparative iron quantities, Romaine lettuce offers 7.9 milligrams of iron per 100 calories, broccoli 3.1 mg, mushrooms 6.4, mung bean sprouts 3.0, black beans 2.2, lentils 2.9, and pumpkin seeds 2.8.

By comparison, beef, per 100 calories, contains only 0.8 mg of iron, chicken 0.6 mg, cod 0.5 mg, and salmon 0.2 mg. Romaine lettuce provides almost ten times more iron per calorie than meat. With all the other fruits and vegetables you eat, you'll get plenty of iron. If you typically have iron deficiencies (anemia), you may want to talk to a doctor knowledgeable about iron sources and iron blockers in your foods, as well as foods critical in iron adsorption.

OTHER PEOPLE'S BIG BUTS

"Yeah, but...everyone in my family is heavy – it's genetic."

If your family is overweight, then the members of your family have adopted poor eating habits passed down from generation to generation. Rarely is anyone overweight because of a genetic problem. The formula for too much weight is quite simple: too many calories in + too few calories out = too much weight.

Genetics may load the gun in some cases, but we pull the trigger with our choices. Whether you have so-called "good" genes or "bad" genes, it's up to you to maximize their potential by the choices you make every day, instead of blaming your parents for your weight issue.

"Yeah, but...my spouse does the food shopping and makes the meals."

Work with the person who prepares the meals. It's very simple to include salads, fruits, and vegetables in your day, along with other foods. Once your intentions and goals become very clear, and you communicate them to your significant other, that person is usually happy to help.

If nothing else, I suggest you have a heart-to-heart talk with that wonderful person in your life who is willing to shop, plan, and prepare meals for you and say something like this: "Honey, I am making a commitment to myself to lose this weight and get my health back on track. Would you be willing to help me out?"

I can't imagine very many people will say no to this question. But, if your honey doesn't have the inclination to help out, no big deal. How hard is it to get your own fruit and salad stuff, stick it in your mouth, and chew? Sometimes if you actually offer to help with the shopping and food preparation, full cooperation is much easier to come by.

"Yeah, but...my family is not doing 10+10 with me, and it's too hard for me to watch them eat my favorite foods while I have to eat a salad."

No question about it. It's difficult to watch people around you eat the foods you love while you choose a different course. But if you follow the three 10+10 rules and eat the good-for-you foods first until you're full, you'll find that the other foods will lose some of their appeal.

Also, keep in mind that you never "have to" eat a salad. If you eat a salad or any other best-for-you foods, it's your choice – one that will get you that much closer to the goals you have created for yourself. If you're feeling deprived and left out, follow the 10+10 rules and eat a salad first, cooked vegetables second, a whole grain or some beans next, and then, if you still can't resist one of your old-time baddies, go ahead and wiggle, if you must!

BIG BUTS BEGONE!

Now that your eyes are wide open to those "yeah, buts" bulleting right toward you, muster all your might and butt those buts head-on, booting them right out of your brain and life – forever. Ah, that's it. They're gone. Doesn't it feel good to be free – free to listen to and follow your own instincts, reclaiming complete responsibility for your own body and direction for your own life? Now what were your guts telling you about 10+10 and you, right before those big buts so rudely interrupted? Oh, yes…

As you were saying, "I can do it. This time, I'm going to get into those pants – no matter what!" And, by golly, you can and will. Now get ready for even more reinforcement, inspiration, and simple direction…coming as soon as the next page with the answer to your single most burning question…

WHAT YOU NOW KNOW…

- Big buts are inevitable; their stopping you from getting into your pants is not.

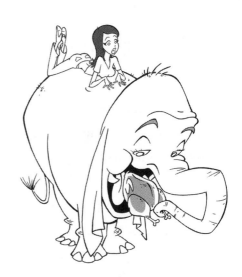

Chapter 11

Protein, Plants, and Pants

"But where do I get my protein?"

- What is protein for?

- How much protein do I need?

- What are my best sources of protein?

No doubt about it. We Americans are confused about food and the three basic nutrients – carbohydrates, fats, and proteins. But of the three, protein seems to be the biggest puzzlement of all. Predictably, the first question people ask me when they start thinking about eating more whole, fresh fruits and vegetables, along with whole grains and beans, is: "If I don't eat as much meat, where do I get my protein?"

After all, it's a fair, logical question, given the thousands of meat-centered meals we've eaten. And it deserves an easy-to-understand, truthful answer.

WHAT IS PROTEIN FOR?

Proteins consist of twenty-two building blocks called amino acids, nine of which must be supplied by outside sources, your foods. Your body makes the others naturally. Amino acids are used to make things like hormones, enzymes, antibodies, cell membranes, and carriers for oxygen in the blood. They're critical for the structure, repair, maintenance, growth, and reproduction of your cells and tissues.

Thanks to the cultural conditioning brought about by the meat, egg, and dairy industries, as well as the protein drink/bar industry, most Americans believe energy is provided by protein. However, the most efficient energy source is not protein at all. The best sources of energy are the carbohydrates found in fresh, whole fruits and vegetables, as well as unrefined grains and beans.

If you compare your body to a car, proteins are the necessary building blocks that form the structure of the engine (structure of your cells). Carbohydrates are the gasoline that runs the engine (your body). Want more pep? Consume more unrefined plant sources of carbohydrates, not more protein.

HOW MUCH PROTEIN DO WE NEED?

"How much," you ask? Not nearly as much as you may think.

Let's keep this simple. Among many other things, we need protein for growth, right? When do we grow the most? From birth to twelve months old. When do we require the most protein? From birth to twelve months old. How much protein is contained in breast milk, the perfect food for rapidly growing babies? About 4.5%. That's all.

Not coincidentally, the World Health Organization recommends that the adult diet consist of 4.5% protein from the total calories consumed. This gets a bit technical, but hang in there with me – this is important. The Institute of Medicine says that the estimated average requirement of protein for a healthy adult is 0.66 grams of protein per kilogram of body weight, per day (.66 g/kg). This is less than half as much as the protein recommended for a baby – 1.5 g/kg a day.

According to these figures, the average requirement each day of protein for women is 38 grams, for men 47 grams. The average American woman over age 20 gets 63.8 grams of protein per day; the average man gets 94.9 grams. In other words, we're eating almost double the protein we need.

So what's wrong with that? Unlike fats and carbohydrates, our bodies cannot store much protein. That means our bodies must somehow get rid of that protein through the liver, kidneys, and urine, forcing our bodies to work overtime. In fact, eating too much protein over time can lead to permanent kidney damage.

Yes, we absolutely need protein for the basic structure of our cells and function of our bodies. No, we don't need nearly as much as we're getting and, in fact, it can be harmful.

I would love to be asked just once, "Dr. Leslie, do you think I'm getting too much protein?"

WHAT ARE MY BEST SOURCES OF PROTEIN?

Now, you may have a clearer idea of how much protein you need, but you're probably still wondering, "Don't I need to eat meat to get protein?"

In a word, no! Of all the food myths out there, the granddaddy myth of all is that you have to eat meat to get your protein. And, not just a little meat, but meat at every meal, every day, every week, every year for life.

The truth is, whole, fresh fruits and vegetables are your best protein sources. They provide plenty of protein, without the depleting fat, cholesterol, and unnecessary calories. I know – a shocker, isn't it? In fact, you're probably just as skeptical as you are shocked. Good. Don't believe me. Seek the facts for yourself. I want you to read, think, read, and think some more. Challenge yourself. Challenge me. This is *your life* (and your pants) we're talking about.

To jumpstart your quest for the truth, here are a few facts about animal- vs. plant-based proteins:

Plant-Based Proteins (fruits/vegetables/grains/beans/nuts/seeds)
- Whole, fresh fruits and vegetables provide all the proteins necessary for you to thrive. Add to them whole grains and beans, and you're filling up on the foods that contain exactly zero animal protein, zero cholesterol, and are usually naturally low in fats – oh, yes, we love that low-fat part.

- All amino acids, whether from plant or animal sources, are equally effective. As long as you get all of your nine essential amino acids, you're good to go. However, the plant protein comes without all the added fat, cholesterol, hormones, and chemicals that come with animal proteins. All of these hidden additions to animal-based foods add piles of calories and make it harder for your body to function correctly and shed pounds.

- The World Health Organization recommends 4.5% protein in your diet. Oranges contain 8%, grapefruit 8%, tomato 16%, Romaine lettuce 36% protein (yes! that much!), spinach 36%, broccoli 33%, cauliflower 26%, corn 11% (who doesn't like corn), potato 8%, carrot 9%, berries 7%, almonds 13%, pumpkin seeds 17%, brown rice 8%, oats 17%, kidney beans 27%, and kale 22%. Are you getting a clearer protein picture?

- According to the American Dietetic Association and many nutrition experts, there's no need to consciously mix and match plant foods to get a so-called "complete protein." Mixing and matching is a myth. As long as you eat a colorful variety of fruits and vegetables, you'll get all of your amino acids without once looking at a chart.

Animal-Based Proteins (meats/dairy/eggs)

- All animal proteins are accompanied by artery-clogging and heart-stopping cholesterol, also linked to leukemia and cancers of the liver, colon, lung, breast, brain, and stomach. And, red meat is not the only baddie for high cholesterol. Read and be amazed at what you choose to pump into your arteries. For a 3.5 oz. serving, beef contains 85 milligrams of cholesterol, chicken 85 mg (just as much as beef!), pork 90 mg, trout 73 milligrams.

- The protein provided by beef, poultry, lamb, pork, wild game, fish, eggs, and dairy products is usually accompanied by excess fat that comes in the animal product. Skinless chicken has 39% fat from total calories, salmon 48% fat, eggs 62%, and cheddar cheese a whopping 73% fat. Fat contributes to many conditions and killer diseases, like heart disease, breast cancer, diabetes, stroke, digestive problems, and obesity.

• According to T. Colin Campbell's book, *The China Study*, animal protein alone, completely separate and distinct from animal fat and cholesterol, may be one of the most toxic substances that we eat. He found a shocking correlation between isolated animal protein and killer diseases, like heart disease, breast cancer, colon cancer, prostate cancer, kidney diseases, and osteoporosis.

I hope this helps make some sense out of the protein debate.

However, if you're still confused, look to nature for some simple logic. How do our largest mammals, elephants, giraffes, horses, and cows develop their great, big muscles and bones and get all their strength and energy? By eating chicken, hamburgers, steak, ham and cheese sandwiches, fish, eggs, and protein drinks? Hardly. They eat plants, and not a huge variety at that. And they certainly don't worry about mixing and matching plant proteins. Are we different from elephants? You bet we are – a whole lot smaller. If they can obtain all the nutrition needed for their huge bodies through plant foods, we can, too.

Meat is a choice, not a need. Make your choice and take responsibility for the consequences of that choice.

WHAT YOU NOW KNOW...

- Proteins are critical for the structure, repair, maintenance, growth, and reproduction of cells and tissues.

- Protein is not the body's preferred energy source, carbohydrates are.

- Plants, even just fruits and vegetables, provide plenty of protein for the human body to thrive (oranges are 8% protein).

- Animal protein is associated with fat, cholesterol, hormones, and chemicals.

- Animal protein may be one of the most toxic, disease-causing substances that we eat.

- When in doubt, look to nature for answers: where do elephants get their protein for great, big muscles?

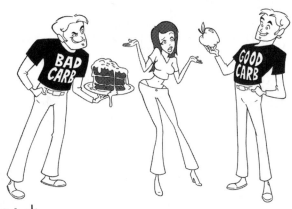

Chapter 12

The 20-Carb Solution into Your Pants

"But don't carbs make me fat?"

- What are carbohydrates?
- What's the difference between good carbs and bad carbs?
- How do you spot the bad guys?

Every time I hear someone say, "I'm trying to stay away from carbs," I'm reminded that the high-protein, low-carb craze changed our culture's climate from carb-clueless to carb-phobic, neither of which has helped us eat any better or weigh any less.

If you remember only one fact about carbohydrates, remember this: carbohydrates are *not* created equally. There are good carbs and bad carbs. Let's separate the good boys from the bad boys so that you know who to hang out with, who to steer clear of, and why.

WHAT ARE CARBOHYDRATES?

Of the three major nutrients, proteins, fats, and carbohydrates, carbo-hydrates provide your body's preferred fuel, the energy that makes your engine purr. With the two exceptions of milk sugar (lactose) and eggs, carbohydrates are found *only* in plants. Created through the process of photosynthesis, carbohydrates are nature's way of capturing the energy of the sun and offering that energy to you in the form of power-packed fruits, vegetables, whole grains, and legumes.

If you break a plant down into its different nutrients – carbohy-drates, proteins, and fats – you find that the biggest hitters for carbo-hydrates are fruits at 90-95%. Vegetables contain 50-90%, grains 65-85%, and legumes 65-75%. That means at least half of almost every plant food powers you with energy.

Take a look at these common carbohydrate-rich, feed-me foods. Broccoli contains 58% carbohydrates, Romaine lettuce 54%, green beans 76%, potatoes 92%, carrots 87%, bean sprouts 64%, spinach 54%, apples 95%, oranges 91%, bananas 92%, kidney beans 70%, and brown rice 85%.

On the other hand, animal products are devoid of carbohydrates, meaning they provide very little or no energy. Eggs contain only 3% carbohydrates, cheese 1%, and all meats (beef, chicken, turkey, pork, lamb) and seafood exactly 0% carbohydrates, the rest fat and protein.

If you're missing the get up and go you used to have, think about how much fuel (how many carbs) you're feeding your engine. Are you eating too many of the depleting foods – meat, cheese, and eggs – that provide little or no energy, and not nearly enough of the energy, feed-me foods – whole, fresh fruits, vegetables, whole grains and legumes? And are the carbohydrates you're getting mostly the depleting "bad boy carbs," as in refined, white sugar and white flour products?

Before discussing the "bad boys," let's look at the importance of the "good carbs." Besides providing energy, carbohydrates are packaged in low-calorie, unrefined plant foods, which boost health, prevent diseases, crush cravings, satisfy your hunger drive, and, of course, promote weight loss. That's precisely why whole, fresh fruits and vegetables are the foundational foods upon which 10+10 is built. It makes perfect sense to add and fill up on these calorie-low, nutrient-dense, energy-packed foods first to get your weight down and build your energy and body up.

Can it be that simple? Just add and fill up on carbohydrate-rich foods: your weight will drop, and your energy will hop? Yes, it's that simple if (that's a great, big *if*) you eat the right carbs.

WHAT'S THE DIFFERENCE BETWEEN GOOD AND BAD CARBS?

As you've probably heard, there are both simple and complex carbohydrates. A simple carbohydrate is made from one or two sugar molecules. When these simple molecules hook together, they form complex carbohydrates, often referred to as starches – and no, starches in this sense are not necessarily the bad guys, as you'll soon see. Your digestive system efficiently breaks down both simple sugars and complex starches and then easily absorbs them to supply you miraculously with unlimited pools of energy.

Don't get stuck on the simple and the complex – those terms have no practical use for you. There are both good and bad simple carbohydrates and good and bad complex carbohydrates, depending upon which food provides them.

For example, whole, fresh fruits provide good-for-you simple carbohydrates, while refined sugars provide bad-for-you simple carbohydrates. Yams provide good-for-you complex carbohydrates, while refined, white flours provide bad-for-you complex carbohydrates. Simply put, the natural sugar that comes with the whole, fresh fruit is good for you, as well as the natural starch in the yam. The unnatural, refined white sugar in sweets is bad for you, as well as its partner-in-crime, refined white flour in baked goodies.

The good carb, bad carb debacle becomes a total non-issue if you eat only whole, fresh plant foods, nature's best sources for good carbs. When you venture into the 20% wiggle room, being carb-savvy will help you make more, better choices, and sometimes even the conscious choice not to eat a favorite food that contains bad carbs (and usually other baddies). Good for you if you make that choice!

What's a Bad Carb?

When whole plant foods are refined – a process that strips away the fibrous outer shell and valuable nutrients – sugars, starches, and void-of-nutrition calories are left. These highly concentrated refined sugars, flours, and grains are used to make processed foods that stock the shelves in grocery stores and fill the American belly with brown-colored white breads, rolls, pasta, muffins, bagels, tortilla shells, cereals, baked goods, cookies, cakes, pies, doughnuts, pastries, crackers, candy, chocolate, ice cream, frozen yogurt, jams, sugary drinks, soft drinks, canned foods, packaged foods, soups, spreads, salad dressings, ketchup, mayonnaise, pickles, spaghetti sauces, even baby foods – and that's certainly not all, folks.

So What?

These refined carbohydrates are the quintessential opposite of getting the most nutrients for your calorie buck. Bad carbs bring with them calories, usually lots of them. No longer are they wrapped neatly in nature's perfect package of vitamins, minerals, enzymes, phytochemicals, antioxidants, all the other micronutrients, as well as colon-sweeping fiber. Filling up on these empty carbs results in calorie overload with zero nutrition. In addition, these bad carbs sadly shove aside your weight warriors and health heroes – whole, fresh fruits and vegetables.

Often after eating nutrient-deficient and high-caloried bad carbs, you won't feel full and satisfied, or you'll get hungry right away. Your body craves the nutrients and energy it didn't get from those empty foods. If you fill up on the feed-me carbs, your hunger drive will be satisfied and your energy reserves restored, thereby warding off cravings.

Along with triggering cravings, bad carbohydrates, which have been stripped of their natural, digestion-slowing fiber, are absorbed too quickly into your blood stream, bombarding your blood with sugar. These sugar surges trigger the pancreas to shoot insulin into the blood stream.

These constant sugar spikes do two things: First, they wear out the pancreas, leading to type 2 diabetes, and second, they add fat to your fat. The body turns the excess sugar it can't use into fat, of all things, and stores it in your fat, the fat you can see and the fat you can't, such as in and around your heart, intestines, all your vital organs, and blood vessels.

Refined Sugars

Even worse, refined sugars make you age before your time. They contribute to wrinkles (yikes!), bagging and sagging skin (double yikes!), clogged arteries as in atherosclerosis, high blood pressure, high cholesterol, high triglycerides, heart disease, type 2 diabetes, some cancers, migraines, kidney damage, asthma, acid stomach, osteoporosis, eczema, arthritis, cataracts, anxiety, fatigue, moodiness, hyperactivity, PMS, and lowered immunity.

Further, as most of us can attest to, white sugar is highly addictive, very difficult to break away from and stay away from. Remember what I said before – when you eat white, refined sugars (basically junk), which are completely empty of nutrients, your body craves more carbs to get those nutrients and energy it desperately needs. That's one of the reasons your rational, thinking mind (it knows better!) says, "No, no, no, I'm not going to eat this," at the exact same moment your misbehaving hand shoves it into your open-like-a-baby-bird mouth. Sound at all familiar?

The best way to deal with these bad boys is to stay away from them. The less you eat, the less you will crave.

Refined Grains

Filling up on white flour products (breads, pastries, bagels, muffins, pastas, tortillas), white rice, instant oats, and other refined grains, along with white sugar, leaves you overfed and undernourished. This triggers increased appetite and cravings for more nutrients, translating into more food, more bad carbs, more calories, more fat, more weight, and more bad self-talk. That's not all. Refined grains, just like white sugar, are major culprits in blood sugar spikes, hypoglycemia, and diabetes. Refined grains may also raise triglycerides (fat in blood), increase risk of heart disease, increase the risk of some cancers (stomach, colorectal, pancreas, breast) and gastro-intestinal disorders like irritable bowel syndrome, and leach hard minerals, like calcium, from your bones, contributing to osteoporosis.

The Whole Famdamly of Baddies

Typically, white sugar and white flour don't like to party alone. They hook up with each other as well as the other baddies, such as salt, oils, fats, chemicals, preservatives, and artificial who-knows-what-else to make up your old-time processed and packaged food faves, all of which deplete you.

HOW DO YOU SPOT THE BAD GUYS?

First of all, go back to the feed-me vs. deplete-me food chart in Chapter 5. The 10+10 super stars in the first box, nature's best, are the whole foods that feed, not deplete, and provide a wealth of good carbohydrates. The first box is a good-carb safety zone. The second box is full of good choices, even though they don't deserve super-star status. This is also a good-carb safety zone.

When you start treading into the third box with some packaged and processed foods, like breads, canned foods, commercial fruit juices, rice or soy milk, or even prepackaged meat substitutes, the bad guys start lurking. Any time a food is altered from its original "whole" state, bad carbs can creep in. Lastly, the entire fourth box is the bad-carb danger zone.

Sometimes bad carbs are sneaky and hard to find. Again, they love to hang out in packs with other bad carbs and other baddies (salt, fats, oils, chemicals, preservatives, flavorings, stabilizers, colorants) in the form of processed foods. Read your labels. Learn this new language, so you can hunt down the bad carbs, along with other baddies. Then make your decision: to eat or not to eat!

Refined sugars are masters of disguise. They can be labeled as sugar, brown sugar, corn syrup, rice syrup, dextrose, glucose, sucrose, lactose, maltose, fructose, dextrin, barley malt, "no sugar added," turbinado, evaporated cane juice, fruit juice concentrate, honey, and maple syrup. In their natural, unrefined states, honey, maple syrup, and molasses may be better choices than refined, white sugars, but they should still be used sparingly. They are concentrated sugars, and those calories come at a premium with almost no nutrients.

White flours are usually easier to spot. The term "wheat flour" for all practical purposes is synonymous with white flour, not *whole* wheat flour. Ninety-nine percent of all breads contain white flour. As a general rule, if bread is not labeled 100% whole wheat, 100% whole grain, or 100% sprouted grain, then white flour lies within. And, even with that 100% on the packaging, be suspicious. Labelers are expert tricksters! Read the label carefully, not just for bad carbs, but also for the other baddies the bad carbs hang out with.

At this point, my personal motto is now very simple: if it has a label, don't eat it. No, I'm not kidding! The only exceptions are raw, unsalted nuts and seeds, but the label has just one ingredient, such as "pumpkin seeds," "sunflower seeds," or "almonds." However, my motto doesn't have to be your motto. Just make sure you know what you're eating before you eat it.

It's important to note that even if bread is 100% whole grain or sprouted grain, bread is still not what I consider a whole grain, as is brown rice, whole barley, millet, or whole oats. No matter how you slice it, bread is a highly processed food, made from the altered fragments of nature's whole grains or sprouts, stripping vital nutrients and leaving a very dense, compromised food that is not pants-friendly.

Breads can also be highly addictive (because of the processed carbs they contain). And, as I've said before, bread always comes with an entourage of ingredients that deplete, not feed. Look for yourself the next time you go grocery shopping. Even the best breads are made with salt, a sweetener, oil, and additives.

Welcome to Club Carb!

You're now an official member of the carb-savvy club (shoot – you've gotten this far in the book, you deserve some recognition). And, just like all carb-savvy club members, your automatic response to your next, "Wow! You look great in those pants. How did you lose weight?" will be:

"I've said goodbye to the bad carbs – no more sweets and white flour goodies for me. I'm filling up on the good carbs found in fresh, whole fruits and vegetables, my true health heroes, weight warriors, and party pants partners. Wanna join us?"

WHAT YOU NOW KNOW...

- Your energy today is sourced by yesterday's 20 or more good carbs you ate yesterday.

- Good carbs are sourced by feed-me, whole plant foods: fresh fruits, fresh vegetables, whole grains, and legumes.

- Bad carbs, empty of nutrition and high in calories, are sourced by refined and processed plant foods, as in white sugar and white flour.

- Read your labels!

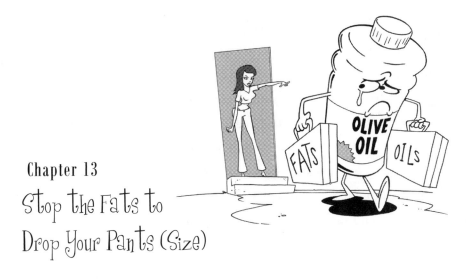

Chapter 13

Stop the Fats to Drop Your Pants (Size)

"But isn't olive oil a good fat?"

- What are fats?

- What's the worst fat?

- What's all the ta-do about good fats/bad fats?

- What's the deal with trans fats and hydrogenated fats?

F-A-T is a three-letter "four-letter" word. And a powerful one at that. F-A-T has the power to sting, to sadden, to madden, to irritate, to frustrate, to incite, to sear, to shame, and to scar. It's a word we'd rather not read, talk, or hear about ever again, and especially not see. But it remains ever-present and heavy in our minds and lives, and for obvious reasons.

As counter intuitive as it may seem, fat is a good thing. We need it – just please, not so much of it. Contrary to the American mentality, "more is better," more fat is not better. In fact, whether it comes from a cow, a fish, a vegetable, a seed, or an olive, too much fat adds fat to our fat. Worse than that, fat is deadly. It's the biggest, "baddest" guy that pulls the trigger in our biggest killers: heart disease, cancers, diabetes, stroke, and atherosclerosis. Further, fat clogs and destroys blood vessels that lead to everywhere – heart, brain, lungs, liver, kidneys, bladder, stomach, small intestine, colon, gall bladder, pancreas, skin, muscles, bones, legs, feet, wrists, hands, eyes, ears, gums, and sexual organs.

Having problems? Strip away the emotions trapped in the layers, make an honest, clear-headed assessment of what you're putting into your body, and then do something about it.

It's time to face your demon: F-A-T.

WHAT ARE FATS?

Fats consist of fatty acids that play a critical role in the structure of cell membranes. When stored, fats also provide usable energy when the body is deprived of its more efficient, preferred energy sources – unrefined carbohydrates. Fat is nature's way of bolstering the chances of survival for human beings in times of food scarcity – not a huge problem in America these days. We may be undernourished, but it's because we're overfed, not underfed.

Basically, there are two kinds of fats – saturated and unsaturated. Saturated fats, solid at room temperature, are found predominantly in animal tissues. Unsaturated fats, liquid at room temperature, are found predominantly in plants, i.e. highly processed, refined oils.

Unsaturated plant fats can be subdivided into two categories: monounsaturated and polyunsaturated. Monounsaturated fats can be found in avocados, most nuts, olive oil, and canola oil. Polyunsaturated fats can be found in vegetable oils, green-leafy vegetables, broccoli, cabbage, corn, avocado, nuts, seeds, grains, legumes, and many other plant foods.

The next fat fact will frizzle your brain's hard drive. Play along with me for a little fat fun.

Guess where almost all needed fats come from? No peeking now. Meat, cheese, vegetable oils, olive oil, or whole plant foods? Knowing how well you know me by now, I'm guessing you guessed whole plant foods. Right? Well, you're wrong! I fooled you! I fooled you! Give it one more try. Where do most of the fats you need come from?

Ready for this? They don't "come from" anywhere – your body makes them! Do you have any idea how fat smart your body is? What's the point for all that agonizing over good fats, bad fats anyway? A big, profitable point for the big, fat fat industry, but no point for you. Quit the fat debate – your body is way smarter than you. It makes almost all the fat it needs from the carbohydrates you eat. Who would have "thunk" it?

What that means to you is this: you need to eat very little fat, and especially *not* added oils (including olive oil) and high fat foods. In fact, if you eat the 10+10 way, you don't need to think about fat at all – your body thinks for you.

Ironic isn't it? No need to think about the consumption of fat, yet fat can easily consume your thinking.

WHAT'S THE WORST FAT?

Etch forever in your mind another very important fact about fat, and the other two macronutrients (proteins and carbs): *Extra cals are not your pals, gals.*

Unrefined carbs, plant proteins, and fats, no matter how good for you, turn bad in a hurry if overeaten. This one pearl of wisdom, if acted upon, can drop the size of your pants in a hurry and keep on dropping…until you're defying gravity – loving the way you look and feel.

Fats, with nine kilocalories per gram – over twice that of proteins and carbohydrates – are the easiest to overeat. And what's the most effective strategy for not overeating, besides the unreliable PAT method (Push Away from the Table)? Get all your feed-me carbohydrates, proteins, and a few fats from the most natural, unadulterated sources as possible – whole plant foods.

The bottom line that affects your bottom's line is this: your body doesn't care where excess calories come from. If you overload and tip the calorie-in part of the calorie-in/calorie-out teeter-totter, your body's job is to do something with those weighty, unneeded, extra calories. Therefore, if your body can't eliminate them, it efficiently turns calories into fat and dumps fat where it can be stored – into your fat cells. And when your fat cells get too fat, your clever body will simply make more fat cells to accommodate the influx of more fat.

Oh, great! Just what we all want – more fat cells, fat cells that do get skinnier with weight loss, but *never* disappear! Isn't that an ugly thought? Once you make a fat cell, that cell is embedded in your hip, thigh, tummy, butt, arm, breast, or chin for life – always ready for that instant refill upon demand. Now that's a legitimate reason to moan out loud.

The worst fat is overeaten fat. If you're going to expend your energy thinking about fat, then think about this the next time you are tempted to overeat: fat goes from your lips to your hips, so get a grip. STOP eating!

WHAT'S ALL THE TA-DO ABOUT GOOD FATS/BAD FATS?

When it comes to fat, most of the time eating even a little is eating too much, except the natural fats that come in whole, unrefined plant foods.

Take *saturated fats,* for instance, found mostly in animal products. There is no good fat/bad fat question here – these are bad fats that break down your body and pack on the pounds. Even a little of something bad is still bad. If a cigarette smoker asked you how many cigarettes were okay to smoke in a day, what would you tell her? Are five okay? How about three? Even one?

Now ask yourself that same question about saturated fats found in these percentages of total calories: beef 67%, chicken 48%, cheddar cheese 73%, egg 62%, salmon 48%, 2% milk 35%. Knowing that saturated fats significantly increase the risk for killers like heart disease, type 2 diabetes, stroke, high blood pressure, as well as lung, breast, prostate, uterine, and colorectal cancers, not to mention being 10, 20, or 50 pounds overweight, how much saturated fat should you eat in a day? None. Period.

(Side note: saturated fats are not to be confused with cholesterol. Cholesterol is a so-called sterol, another important component in the cell structure. Your body produces all the cholesterol it needs. When cholesterol, found in all animal products, is consumed, it accumulates as a waxy-like substance along with fat inside the blood vessels, making plaque, or unstable, "burstable," pimple-like sores, and diseases right along with it. Plant foods have exactly zero cholesterol.)

Back to fats. Then there are those *polyunsaturated* and *monounsaturated fats.* Because all those clear, bottled oils are extracted from plants, they must be good fats, right? Wrong. On the contrary, these refined oils are bad fats, too. Yes, as much as this will shake up Queen

Olive's kingdom, even cold-pressed, organic, triple-extra virgin olive oil is bad for you. Why?

Follow this simple logic. If your body makes almost all the fats it needs, then it serves no purpose whatsoever to add more fat to the ready-made fat, especially a highly concentrated, refined fat that comes without any nutrition. Added oils offer you one thing only: calories, and those calories come with a fat price tag – more fat. And, it just so happens that between 14 and 17 percent of olive oil is saturated. How can extra calories and saturated fat possibly be good for you, no matter how loud the cry from Queen Olive's loyal subjects?

Besides adding extra calories, refined oils reduce the ability of blood vessels to dilate (expand) and cause the blood cells to get sticky and clump together, thereby reducing their ability to carry oxygen to your body, including your brain. This lack of oxygen makes you sleepy after a fat-laden meal. Oils, like all unnecessary fats, also contribute to the proliferation of cancer and to the build up of heart attack- and stroke-causing plaque in blood vessels, causing cardiovascular disease, stroke, hypertension, type 2 diabetes, gallstones, kidney stones, and obesity. Furthermore, when oils are heated, whether fried or baked, they produce cancer-causing free radicals.

Caldwell B. Esselstyn, Jr., M.D., a heart specialist and the author of *Prevent and Reverse Heart Disease,* who has been unbelievably successful in reversing heart disease in very seriously heart-ill people, states an excellent case for the elimination of all processed oils, including olive oil and high-fat foods. He will not work with anyone who won't follow his protocol of no added oils, no added fats, no meat, and no high-fat foods. That's one of the reasons he gets results.

Two "Good Fats"

Goodness. And you thought you were doing your body a huge health favor by being so particular about eating all that olive oil! So, if the lovely Queen Olive isn't a member of the good fat family, then who is?

Meet linoleic and alpha-linoleic fatty acids, two essential poly-unsaturated fats. The word "essential," in this case, means that because your body lacks the ability to make these fatty acids, you must get them from your foods.

You are probably familiar with the buzz words omega-6 fats and omega-3 fats. Linoleic is an omega-6 fat, and alpha-linoleic an omega-3 fat. I will skip the details of the omegas here and how it's the ratio (which is controversial) between the omega-6s and the omega-3s that appears to be important. For the most part, those details will not help you lose weight. Whether a fat is called saturated, polyunsaturated, monounsaturated, omega-6, omega-3, or Queen Olive, if you add fat to already-made fat, no matter who tells you what, that fat is a bad fat and shows up on you.

Instead of trying to remember all the pet names for fats and what they mean, it's a lot easier to remember the best sources for those two essential fatty acids that you need: whole plant foods. What a surprise! Yes, you can get one or both of these good fats in these concentrat-ed oils – flax seed oil, canola oil, soybean oil, olive oil, fish oil – but again, those oils come with only fat and calories without the advantage of being wrapped up with nutrients auto-packaged in whole foods. I remind you once again, you want the most nutrition for your calorie buck and eating pure fat is certainly *not* the way to do that.

The whole, plant foods that are richest in linoleic acids are sun-flower, pumpkin, and sesame seeds, walnuts, butternuts, soybeans, and corn; in alpha-linoleic acid, dark, green-leafy vegetables, broccoli, sea-weeds, ground flax seeds, soybeans, walnuts and butternuts. If you eat a varied diet of mostly whole, fresh fruits and vegetables, along with whole grains, beans, and a significantly lesser amount of raw nuts and seeds, you can get all the essential good fats without consciously having to choose special foods high in those particular fats. And, lose weight besides.

According to the pioneer in whole, plant-based diets, John Mc-Dougall, M.D., author of several books, including *The McDougall Plan – 12 Days to Dynamic Health*, points out that a plant-based diet provides all the essential fats we need. George Eisman, registered dietician, author of *The Most Noble Diet*, tells us that a diet rich in just whole fruits and vegetables offers an average of 5% calories from essential fatty acids, more than the 3% the government recommends.

To give you a feel for how much fat plant foods offer, oranges contain 2% fat, apples 4%, bananas 4%, berries 10%, brown rice 7%, whole wheat bread 5%, almonds 74%, kidney beans 3%, broccoli 9%, and Romaine lettuce 10% – yes, even lettuce has fat!

Once again, nature proves that she is wiser than her human charges. If you fill up on nature's feed-me, best-for-you foods – whole plant foods, with the emphasis on fresh, fruits and vegetables – you can cut the internal and external chatter about which foods provide which nutrients. Nature has done all that higher nutrient math for you!

WHAT ABOUT TRANS FATS AND HYDROGENATED FATS?

As if vegetable oils and animal fats aren't bad enough for your body and boggling enough for your mind, the most notorious fat villains of all, although quietly subversive, are next to hit the scene: trans fats and hydrogenated fats.

Simply put, *trans fats*, or altered fats, are sometimes referred to as synthetic saturated fats. They cause the same destruction as both unsaturated and saturated fats, leading to higher cholesterol levels, heart disease, and some cancers. Further, they compromise the immune system (fighting diseases), nerve system (the coordination and control of all functions in your body), and metabolic system (how well your body can metabolize or use the foods and calories you eat). Trans fats also love to congregate in adipose tissues – your fat.

In Harvard Medical School's Nurses Health Study of 85,095 women, as reported in *The Lancet*, 1993, both saturated and trans fats increased coronary heart disease, but nurses who consumed considerable amounts of trans fat faced an even higher risk of heart attack than nurses who ate a lot of saturated fat.

Hydrogenated or partially hydrogenated fats are liquid oils processed into a solid or semi-solid state using high heat and hydrogen gas, as in margarines and vegetable shortenings. What's the purpose of hydrogenation? To add creamy smooth texture to some foods and to extend the shelf life of products. Sadly, the tradeoff for an artificially-contrived longer shelf life could be a shorter life for you.

Trans fats result from the hydrogenation of oils. If a food contains hydrogenated or partially hydrogenated fats, it automatically contains trans fats as well. Experts agree that trans fats and hydrogenated fats should be eliminated, not just avoided. And they seem to be everywhere! Read your labels and do yourself a huge favor – don't eat the foods that contain trans fats and hydrogenated fats.

Look out for their local hang-outs:

- Almost all commercial breads (it's true – see for yourself)

- Fried foods, as in French fries, onion rings, chicken, fish

- Stick and tub margarines

- Butter substitutes

- Mayonnaise

- Shortening

- Spreads

- Dips

- Chips

- Crackers

- Cereals

- Salad dressings

- Peanut butter

- Chocolate

- Candy, including even some hard candies

- Pizza

- Processed foods

- Packaged foods

- Packaged snack foods

- Packaged energy/protein bars

- Vegetarian/vegan processed foods like veggie/soy-type burgers

- Pre-made meals, like frozen dinners

- Pre-made diet meals

- Baked goods, like rolls, muffins, bagels, biscuits

- Baked goodies, like cookies, cakes, pies, desserts of all kinds

- Microwaved popcorn

Tips to avoid trans fats and hydrogenated fats:

1. Read labels and learn what the words mean.

2. Hunt for foods that contain <u>no</u> "vegetable shortening," "hydrogenated" or "partially hydrogenated oils." Good luck!

3. Foods labeled "cholesterol free" or "low cholesterol," "low saturated fat," or "made with vegetable oil" may still contain trans fats.

4. Look for "no trans fats" or "saturated fat free."

WHAT YOU NOW KNOW...

- Fat is a major nutrient needed for health.

- The worst kind of fat is too much fat.

- Your body makes almost all the fats you need (two exceptions which can be sourced by plants).

- How much saturated fat and refined oils (including olive oil) should you eat? None.

- How much trans fat and hydrogenated fat should you eat? None.

- Whole plant foods provide all the essential fats you need.

And the simplest, most brilliant fat fact of all: *The fat you eat is the fat you wear!* Are those few seconds of pleasure when fat goes down worth the pain of where it ends up?

But for all this discussion about fat, let's not forget that with 10+10, you can wiggle a bit and still lose the jiggle. Just don't wiggle too much, or the jiggle will keep you out of those pants.

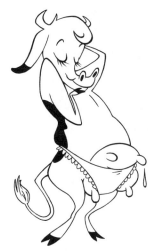

Chapter 14

Dairy's Dirty Underpants

"If I don't drink milk, where do I get my calcium?"

- Please, oh Pleeeease Don't Take My Cheese! (A personal story)

- Airing Dairy's Dirty Underpants

- Revealing Calcium's Secret Stash

ood is addictive – as we all can attest. Whether it's a physical, mental, emotional, conditional, cultural, or all-of-the-above addiction makes no difference. We're hooked, and that's why it's so tough to leave certain foods alone – no matter how much we try to think or talk ourselves out of them.

Following the 10+10 rule of adding the best foods first – whole, fresh fruits and vegetables – really does cut cravings for the goodies but baddies, but they still can call to us with inexplicable urgency and power at the most unexpected times.

For some of us, it's sweets that woo; for others, it's salt. It can be greasy chips we choose or diet pop we gulp. Bread soothes, meat rules. Countless combos connive to command and control. And let's not forget the dark devil himself, a seductive master who leaves us weak in the knees and vacant of sense…chocolate. Everyone has at least one weak spot when it comes to bad foods.

One demon that lures with irresistible magnetism is dairy – milk (with cookies, of course), ice cream, yogurt, cream in your coffee, whipped cream, butter, and the biggest dairy seducer of all, cheese.

Dancing with the dairy demon spells: D-A-N-G-E-R. But that couldn't include our beloved <gulp> cheese, could it?

PLEASE, OH PLEEEEASE DON'T TAKE MY CHEESE!

Excuse me while I indulge in a little whine with my cheese.

As you now know, in 10+10 you think about which foods you "get to" add, not which foods you "have to" give up. So don't panic when I talk about my own struggle to stay away from cheese.

Although I'm referring to cheese, cheese can easily be interchanged with your food nemesis, whether it's sugar, salt, meat, bread, pizza, fast foods, junk foods, fried foods, diet pop, or heaven forbid, all of the above.

There's no denying, no matter what strategies we use to lose weight, certain foods stubbornly cling to us harder than others. Over time, as I shifted my food day more and more toward whole plant foods, I gradually worked all those other bad boys out of my life. But that cheese was my love, and my demon. It was simple – if it was around, I couldn't resist – I ate it. And I, as a responsible, decision-making adult, tried to sneak it into my grocery cart (as if I could fool myself) to make sure it was around. As far as I was concerned, I could live without any other food. But life without cheese? No way. No how. Wouldn't go there.

That would mean life without Canadian sharp, pizza, tacos, enchiladas, lasagna, macaroni and cheese, fettuccini Alfredo, crackers and cheese, bleu cheese dressing, veggies with cheese, cheesy sauces and dishes, and my best college buddy of all – orange cheddar smeared with mayo between two pieces of brown-colored, white bread.

I was adamant. I had given up so much – I was not going to give up cheese, even cutting back was a struggle. And then…I did it.

It didn't happen in a day – more like 3000 days, without exaggeration. (I know – that's over eight years!) I was that emotionally and physically attached to cheese. Somehow, one painful baby step at a time, with hundreds of crash-booms in between, I weaned myself from my binkie – wailing the whole time. No, there was nothing brave or noble about poor me and my perceived pain.

Goodbye sniff, sniff, sniff

I made the commitment to work away from cheese for three reasons. First, intellectually, I knew it wasn't good for me with its fat, cholesterol, salt, dyes, and chemicals. Second, eating cheese was incongruent to what I believed and was teaching, dinging my integrity. Third, I hated the fact that cheese had such a hold on me – it made me feel, well, out of control. Being addicted to anything is a horrible, helpless feeling.

I knew that dairy products were strongly associated with many physical problems, from minor nuisances like head congestion and colds, to major diseases like cancer and heart disease. But I didn't know that I was the walking, talking poster girl for dairy's darker side of that ubiquitous white mustache.

As ridiculous as it sounds, I was clueless about how dairy had performed its dirty work on me my whole life – from screaming earaches and doubling-over stomachaches as a kid to headachy sinus pressure and that constant sniffing as an adult. When I at long last ripped myself away from cheese, I finally "got milk" and how milk had "got me."

After being off cheese for several weeks, I noticed that something was missing – the sniffing. It was gone.

The sniff and I had been best buds since birth. As my constant companion, it was with me when I first woke up in the morning, sniff, sniff, sniff, and on and off throughout the day – every day. It was one of those things that I had lived with so long; I had no idea it wasn't supposed to be there.

But when cheese disappeared, the most miraculous thing happened – my head got clear – first time ever. Ah, so that's what noses were for – to breathe air in and to breathe air out. After a lifetime of blowing, I was blown away. I thought noses were built like broken, leaky faucets – with an incessant drip, drip, drip, drip.

And the sniff was not the only thing that had vanished – so did my sinus headaches, as well as those earaches and stomachaches, which had been less frequent as an adult but still nagged me. And my energy kicked up a notch or two. It was the first time I had personally experienced that old adage I had repeated so many times: "You are what you eat." Life without cheese was distinctly different from life with cheese. At the age of forty something, I finally knew what it was like to feel good.

The worst part about my blind refusal to connect those very distinct dots between cheese and me is that I got my own kids hooked on cheese, adding to my youngest daughter's lifelong struggle with weight. Our favorite cheddar cheese was almost 75% fat! How could that be good for you? And I was giving that to the loves of my life – my children! What was I thinking?

That's the whole point – I wasn't. I was the all-American robo-eating-food-fixing machine – eating and fixing exactly what I had been pre-programmed to eat and fix – even though I knew better. I taught this stuff for cryin' out loud. THAT made me furious at myself – after I finally pried my eyes open!

AIRING DAIRY'S DIRTY UNDERPANTS
Milky White Lies

Americans were raised to believe that milk represents purity and goodness. Milk, whether from mama, a formula, or a cow, is our first gut-level connection with comfort, warmth, safety, and love. That connection is nature's way of making babies suckle – ensuring its survival. I'm quite sure nature did not intend for us humans to suckle lifelong. Yet, we sophisticated, smart Americans adamantly accept that suckling milk and eating its products are not only natural and normal, but necessary for life itself. We're so arrogant and self-righteous about our beliefs that we assume the whole world follows our lead.

But it's time to come down from our lofty perch and mingle with some basic truths. The fact is, about 65% of the adults on the planet don't drink milk, and lo and behold, their bones don't crumble and their teeth don't fall out of their heads because of it.

Yet, America's decree from yesteryear (and still today) was loud and clear: you must drink three glasses of milk a day for strong bones and teeth. That's what everyone believed – teachers, doctors, experts, government officials, friends, your mother – and you too. Milk's looming stature was bulked up not just by repetitious rhetoric, but by milk's constant presence in our day-to-day lives – that glass of milk for dinner, cookie and milk treats at a friend's house, the ubiquitous waxed boxes on every hospital and school lunch tray.

Our minds were completely white-washed by that white liquid legend, leaving no room for question. Milk was a natural. And if your fifth grade mind worked anything like mine, it made sense – after all, the white in milk must make our teeth and bones white, too. (What can I say? I was only ten.)

How could a whole culture get lost in a sea of such "udder" nonsense?

Dirty Underwear

Let's dig into dairy's dirty laundry, expertly hidden beneath the cloak of white mustaches on famous, marketable faces.

FACT: Adult human beings are the only mammals that drink milk after they are weaned (and another mammal's milk at that). That in itself should have aroused an inkling of suspicion. Cows' milk is nature's perfect food – for baby cows who can double their weight in 47 days, four times faster than a human baby, and can gain up to 600 pounds in a year – but certainly not for us humans when 65% (or more) of us are battling weight, as well as 25% of our children. Nature is very wise, although we often ignore her guidance. She made sure all mammals provide the perfect food for their own babies, not for the babies of another species. Only human milk is perfectly formulated for humans – and only baby humans at that.

However, the Dairy Council is correct with its relentless, unconscionable message. "Milk has something for everybody." After getting intimate with milk's dirty underpants, you'll agree that milk and its whole family have many "somethings" for one and all:

- **Saturated fat** – Just two of those three 12-ounce glasses of whole milk a day that we all grew up believing we had to drink, and perhaps still do, contain as much saturated fat as a Big Mac. Saturated fat clogs up blood vessels and kills, as in heart attacks, hypertension, stroke, diabetes, and breast, prostate, uterine, and colon cancers. But we all know the evils of fat. We may not know, however, that whole milk derives about 50% of its total calories from saturated fat. Low-fat milk (1% to 2%) is 24% to 35% saturated fat; and even skim milk is 4% to 7% saturated fat. As for cheddar cheese, it's a whopping 74% fat. And, of course, what else does the saturated fat in dairy products do besides give us diseases? It makes us fat.

- **Cholesterol** – Cholesterol is one of the biggest contributors to heart disease and strokes. The inevitable build up of cholesterol is the direct consequence of consuming cholesterol, sourced in high quantities by all animal products, especially the big, bad cow. Cheddar cheese, for instance, contains 27 mg, yogurt 21 mg, and whole milk 22 mg. As John McDougall, M.D., says in "The McDougall Newsletter" (May 2003, Vol. 2 No. 5), milk is like liquid beef when it comes to cholesterol and saturated fat.

According to the ongoing Framingham Heart Study, the largest heart study of all time, virtually no one gets heart attacks if they have a cholesterol level of 150 or below. The average cholesterol level in the U.S. is 210. For vegetarians 161, for vegans (no meat, dairy, or other animal products) 133.

- **Milk sugar or lactose** – About 70% of world is thought to be allergic to the sugar in milk (lactose), causing digestive disturbances, as in indigestion, gas, stomachaches, constipation, and/or diarrhea. In fact, the majority of Americans are lactose intolerant: 90-100% of Asian Americans, 95% of Native Americans, 65-70% of African Americans, 50-60% of Hispanic Americans, and 10% (or more) of Caucasians. Maybe you are too, just like me.

- **Milk protein (casein)** – The protein in milk wreaks havoc in the human body. Milk protein causes "little problems," like extra mucous (snotty noses), colds, fatigue, sinus headaches, sinus infections, earaches, sore throats, tonsillitis, constipation, stomach upsets, allergies, asthma, bronchitis, dermatitis, psoriasis, eczema, bedwetting, pneumonia, irritability, hyperactivity, mood swings, PMS, depression, and muscle pain.

  However, this protein is also linked with big problems such as autoimmune diseases like type 1 diabetes, lupus, rheumatoid arthritis, and multiple sclerosis, as well as heart disease, Parkinson's, Crohn's disease, ulcerative colitis, autism, depression, schizophrenia, injured blood vessels, arteritis that leads to diseased blood vessels or atherosclerosis, iron deficiency anemia, hormone-fed and/or fat-fed cancers, as in prostate, breast, uterine, lung, colon, ovarian, kidney, and pancreatic.

- **Contaminants** – Milk is not so pure. It's the potential hiding place for lots of invisible nasties:

- Bacteria – listeria (usually in cheeses made from milk), salmonella, E. coli, staphylococci, tuberculosis, and Mycobacterium paratuberculosis, which may be related to Crohn's disease.

- Viruses – viruses known to cause leukemia and lymphoma – the incidence of leukemia in people increases with the increased consumption of milk.

- Viruses – 40% of beef herds are infected with the bovine (cow) AIDS virus and 64% with bovine leukemia virus. Can the bovine viruses jump the species barrier to humans as it does to other animals like sheep, goats, and chimpanzees? It is not thought so, but why take the chance?

Does pasteurization kill dangerous microorganisms? Yes, but it is not 100% foolproof – some slip by. Why take the chance?

- **Pesticides and herbicides** – The environmental toxins that cows get from their plant foods go into the milk they produce. Cows' milk isn't the only toxic stew, so is mother's milk. In a study by the Environmental Defense Fund of 1400 lactating women in forty-six states, widespread pesticides were found in breast milk. Pesticide levels in the breast milk of women who ate meat and dairy were twice as high as levels in vegetarians' breast milk. Makes you think, doesn't it?

- **Hormones** – The production of insulin-like growth hormones (IGF-1) is stimulated in your body by the consumption of animal products, especially dairy products. Injected artificial growth hormones, used to stimulate the production of cow's milk, increases the IGF-1 in cows that, in turn, increases the IGF-1 in their milk. Note: As Dr. John McDougall reports, pasteurization does not destroy IGF-1. More so than in any other food, the IGF-1 in milk raises the level of IGF-1 in you.

So what? IGF-1 promotes the growth of cancer! As T. Colin Campbell, PhD, says in *The China Study*, the correlation between the marker IGF-1 in the blood stream and prostate cancer is just as strong as the correlation between cholesterol and heart disease. The other hormone-fed cancers that are significantly linked to IGF-1 in milk are breast, lung, and colon cancers. Take heed.

- **Antibiotics** – Because artificial hormones overwork cows' udders to make more milk, the incidents of udder infections is increased by 50% to 70%. Antibiotics are used to treat those infections. Yes, residues from antibiotics end up in the milk you drink. But, infections lead to even nastier stuff. Get this...

- **Pus** – When a cow has an infected udder, pus ends up in the milk. Yes, you read it right – that's pus! Ick! And double ick! At any given time, judging by how common udder infections are, you have a 50% or greater chance of eating cow pus in that glass of creamy, smooth, pure white liquid you're putting up to your lips! Don't worry though. The pus patrol keeps the situation under control. In accordance with the Federal Pasteurized Milk Ordinance, our government won't allow any more than 180 million pus cells for one 8 ounce glass of milk!

The Dairy-Disease Connection

In case it got lost in the laundry, there's a strong connection between dairy products and cancer. The saturated fat, cholesterol, milk protein, milk sugar, and hormones contribute in varying degrees to different killer cancers: prostate, breast, uterine, colon, lung, kidney, ovarian, pancreas, lymphoma, and leukemia, and I'm sure there's more.

The American Cancer Society's number one recommendation for the prevention of cancer: eat more plant-based foods (what a surprise!). The American Cancer Society's second recommendation for the prevention of cancer: eat fewer animal-based foods. The information is out there – it's time to listen!

Other dairy-linked diseases and conditions are: heart disease, stroke, types 1 and 2 diabetes, hypertension, Parkinson's, Crohn's, ulcerative colitis, irritable bowel syndrome, multiple sclerosis, lupus, atherosclerosis, rheumatoid arthritis, sinusitis, eczema, sniffing, and the list goes on.

So there you have it – America's pure and perfect, lily-white dream drink shaken up and turned upside down to reveal what lurks hidden beneath – it's anything but clean underpants.

The next time you get the urge, remember the disease-causing, fat-lovin' chemical cocktail you're choosing to put into your body – pus and all. Drink up! And don't forget to make that three a day.

Oh, dear, here it comes – one, two, three – all together now with one gigantic "yeah, but." "Yeah, but if I don't drink milk or eat cheese or yogurt, where do I get my calcium?" I'm so glad you asked because I'm ready to answer that excellent question.

REVEALING CALCIUM'S SECRET STASH

I can answer your calcium questions in just three little sentences.

1. Yes, we certainly do need calcium.

2. No, dairy products for all of the above reasons, and more, are not our best sources of calcium.

3. Yes, fresh, whole fruits and vegetables, with whole grains and beans to boot, are our ideal sources of calcium.

And, if I had to add one more comment it would be this: In the U.S., the key to the calcium balance in the body is not calcium intake (the American diet provides more than enough calcium). It's staying away from the foods and substances that leach calcium out of the body. Osteoporosis, the real concern behind your calcium questions, is not caused by calcium deficiency, or not taking in enough calcium as commonly thought. It is caused by calcium imbalance when too much calcium is being leached from the bones due to what you eat or drink.

That's a lot to take in, so I've answered some of your questions to help clear the calcium and osteoporosis confusion.

Question: How big a problem is osteoporosis in the U.S.?

Answer: Fifty-five percent of all Americans will get osteoporosis. One in two women and one in four men over the age of fifty will suffer an osteoporosis-related fracture in her or his lifetime. Of the people who fracture their hips, twenty-four percent die from that affliction within a year. Twenty percent of adults admitted to nursing homes because of hip fractures never get out. Six months after a hip fracture, only fifteen percent of hip fracture patients can walk across a room unaided.

Question: Do the countries that consume the most dairy products have the least amount of osteoporosis and fractures?

Answer: In a word, no. Interestingly enough, the countries with the highest consumption of dairy products have the highest hip fracture rate and the worst bone health. Those countries are: United States, New Zealand, Sweden, Finland, and England. On the other hand, South Africa, Hong Kong, and Singapore, which consume the most whole plant foods and the least meat and dairy products, have far fewer bone fractures caused by osteoporosis.

Rural China consumes one-half the calcium consumed by Americans, yet it reports one-fifth fewer hip fractures than Americans, as stated by John Robbins in *The Food Revolution* and further substantiated by T. Colin Campbell, PhD, in *The China Study*. Another example, American women drink 30 to 32 times more cows' milk than women in New Guinea, but Americans endure 47 times the hip fractures.

One study showed that the South African Bantu women, who consume only between 250 and 350 mg of calcium, give birth to an average of nine children, breast feed each child from one to two years, develop almost no osteoporosis. They consume no dairy products and eat primarily plant foods.

Question: But how can that be? I thought milk/dairy was supposed to build strong bones and teeth.

Answer: Oh, yes, and so did we all, and in fact, most of us still do. Do the research and answer your own question – they're *your* bones we're talking about. The studies and experts tell a different story from the fairy-tale cow's tale we were told:

- "There is virtually no evidence that drinking two or three glasses of milk a day reduces the chances of breaking a bone." – Walter C. Willet, Chairman of the Department of Nutrition, Harvard School of Public Health.

- A large, 12-year study of 78,000 nurses sponsored by Harvard found no evidence that drinking more milk reduced osteoporosis or bone fracture. In fact, women who drank two or more glasses of milk a day suffered more fractures.

- A study on post menopausal women, published in the *American Journal of Clinical Nutrition*, concluded that women who drank 1400 mg/day of skim milk (3-8 oz. glasses) lost significantly more bone mass than the non milk-drinking women. Ironically, this study was funded by none other than the National Dairy Council. It was not the conclusion the dairy industry was looking for or advertised.

- In 2005, Harvard School of Public Health researched all studies regarding the consumption of milk and its byproducts. It found no evidence supporting the notion that dairy products prevented osteoporosis, much less three glasses of milk a day. It did find, however, that those three glasses of low-fat milk (over 300 calories a day) contributed to overweight and obesity problems, and dairy products were linked to increase risk of ovarian and prostate cancer. Furthermore, due to lactose intolerance, millions of Americans couldn't eat even a little dairy without symptoms of stomach aches, gas, or other digestive problems.

- Robert M. Kradjian, M.D., reviewed over 500 articles published in the scientific, medical literature regarding milk. As he said, "They were only slightly less than horrifying. None of the authors spoke of cow's milk as an excellent food, free of side effects…The main focus of the published reports seems to be intestinal colic, intestinal irritation, intestinal bleeding, anemia, allergic reactions in infants and children, as well as infections such as salmonella…fear of viral infections with bovine leukemia virus or an AIDS-like virus."

Question: If dairy products are not the ideal sources of calcium, what foods are?

Answer: Unrefined plant foods contain all the minerals you need, including calcium. Nature is so smart. Where does calcium come from? The soil. Calcium is dissolved in water and absorbed by plants. Plants transform inedible, unusable calcium from the soil into usable calcium needed by all mammals. Eating plants is the most direct way of getting calcium, and without the fat, cholesterol, animal protein, milk sugar, hormones, antibiotics, and other toxins that come in dairy products.

Again, listen to what the experts tell us.

- According to John Robbins in *Food Revolution*, a survey conducted on diet and hip fractures in 33 countries found "'an absolutely phenomenal correlation'" between eating plant foods and bone strength. The more plants eaten – especially fruits and vegetables – the stronger the bones and the fewer the fractures. The reverse was also true: the more animal foods, the weaker the bones and the more the fractures.

- In *The China Study*, T. Colin Campbell, PhD, professor of nutritional biochemistry at Cornell University, compared the contents of an animal-food combination to a comparable plant food combination. The animal combo was made of equal parts of beef, pork, chicken, and whole milk while the plant combo was made of equal parts of tomatoes, spinach, lima beans, peas, and potatoes. The plant-based foods contained 545 mg of calcium while the animal-based foods contained 252 mg of calcium.

Question: Exactly how much calcium is provided by specific plant foods?

Answer: Here are some plant calcium numbers, sourced by the U.S. Department of Agriculture and *Becoming Vegan* by Brenda Davis, R.D. and Vesanto Melina, M.S., R.D.:

1 cup broccoli – 62 mg

1 sweet potato – 76 mg

1 cup Romaine lettuce – 20 mg

1 cup kale – 94 mg

½ cup green beans – 28 mg

1 navel orange – 60 mg

1 apple – 10 mg

1/2 cup strawberries – 10 mg

¼ cantaloupe – 15 mg

10 figs – 140 mg

¼ cup almonds – 79-115 mg

2 tbs. flax seed – 39 mg

¼ cup sunflower seeds – 40 mg

1 cup kidney beans – 62 mg

1 cup lentils – 38 mg

1/2 cup brown rice – 10 mg

Question: Do I have to consciously eat certain plant foods to make sure I get all of my calcium?

Answer: No, a variety of all plant foods offers you plenty of calcium.

Question: How much calcium do I need in a day?

Answer: The World Health Organization recommends 400 to 500 mg of calcium a day for 50-year-olds and older, while research substantiates the need for only 150-200 mg. Compare that figure to the U.S. government's artificially hiked recommendation, which ranges from 1000 to 1500 mg/day. It's impossible to figure out where that over inflated figure came from (unless the dairy and calcium people had a say).

No matter how much calcium we take in through our foods or tablets, we can only absorb about 500 milligrams a day. The average vegan (no animal products) takes in about 627 mg of calcium per day – plenty!

Question: Do I get osteoporosis from not getting enough calcium?

Answer: Osteoporosis is actually the result of "negative calcium balance" in the body, which means more calcium goes out of the body than comes in, and that typically goes on for decades before showing up as osteoporosis. In the U.S., we get plenty of calcium. The big concern is what we're eating that leaches the calcium out of our bones, dissolving them – and not just right now but what we've been eating our entire lives.

Question: What are the critical years for determining whether I will get osteoporosis or not?

Answer: For a woman, her thirties set the stage for whether she will get osteoporosis; for a man, his forties. It has to do with how much bone mass you build up by this stage of your life. By the time you know you have osteoporosis, even through the most modern testing, you're bones have been dissolving a very long time.

Question: What are the biggest thieves that steal calcium from your bones, causing a "negative" calcium balance?

Answer: Animal protein, sugar, salt, caffeine, alcohol, soft drinks, smoking, and certain drugs, like aluminum-containing antacids (yes, even with calcium added), antibiotics, diuretics, steroids, and chemotherapy. Considering how much you've overloaded your body with some of these day in and day out for most of your life, it's no mystery why you're losing your bones.

Question: What do these calcium thieves have in common?

Answer: Calcium thieves are "acid-producing" foods that make the body more acid. A healthy body is more alkaline. The body neutralizes acidity by pulling the calcium (remember from chemistry class that calcium is a base) out of the bones, which we then proceed to pee out. No surprise – fruits and vegetables are alkaline in nature and can neutralize this acidity. How dangerous is an acid PH in your body? Cancer thrives in an acid environment.

Question: What is the biggest, baddest calcium robber of all?

Answer: Animal protein – beef, chicken, turkey, pork, lamb, fish, shellfish, milk, cheese, yogurt, ice cream, sour cream, cottage cheese, eggs. If you recall, what are proteins made of? Amino acids – as in *acids*. That's a big clue!

Question: What can I do to build my bones up?

Answer: Weight-bearing exercise, like walking, along with the sun's Vitamin D, are very important for stronger bones and muscles.

Question: How much walking should I do to improve my bone health?

Answer: As reported in the *Journal of the American Medical Association* (Nov. 14, 2002), data collected from 61,000 women in the Harvard's Nurses' Health Study showed that if you walk just four hours a week, your risk of hip fracture is reduced by 40%. Hey, that's not much walking at all for the reward of good, strong bones (and everything else)! But don't stop there – this is one of those cases if a little is good, more is better. (More about exercise in Chapter 15.)

Question: At what age is it too late to build up bone strength?

Answer: It's never too late. As long as you are breathing and you can move, you can start building strength.

Question: Do I need to take calcium tablets to get enough calcium?

Answer: This issue is very controversial, as well as a huge money making monster. But my common sense says "No!" if you eat the 10+10 way, unless there are unusual extenuating circumstances. Nature provides you with plenty of calcium – just eat your 10+10 – it's a no brainer and cheaper!

Question: It's a lot to take in. I'm still so confused.

Answer: You're right – it *is* confusing. For a moment, forget all the facts I just shared with you and look to nature for some answers. She's a whole lot smarter than we are. And then, use your own common sense. Where do milking cows and our large, adult mammals, like elephants, horses, giraffes, and apes get their calcium for their big, strong bones and teeth? Certainly not from milk, cheese, or yogurt! They get all the calcium they need from the most direct source – plant foods. If they can, so can we.

Milk's a Choice, Not a Necessity

Now that you have a good idea what lurks beneath the surface of that stiff, upper, white lip, you are fortified with every rational reason to kiss milk and its kin goodbye forever. For me, it boiled down to one very simple question: to sniff or not to sniff?

Your choice could be that simple too: big-girl panties or pretty bikinis?

Do I still miss cheese? Absolutely, even after years without it. Some things never change. Will you miss your feel-good favorites once you let them go? Absolutely. And will knowing all the facts automatically wipe away our passions? Not at all. I still love the stuff and because I know myself well, I follow this motto: I trust myself, but I don't tempt myself.

I keep a safe distance (miles and miles) between cheese and me at all times. I just never know when it could get a mind of its own and fly directly into my open-like-a-baby-bird mouth, at the precise time I'm chanting, "No, no, no, yes, yes, yes, yum, yum, yum, more, more, more, guilt, guilt, guilt, don't care. I'm gonna eat it anyway."

At first, you may think giving up certain foods is nothing short of sacrificial. But with a clear commitment, sustained effort, and the grace of time, that supreme sacrifice transforms into a supreme gift: freedom from food addiction and imprisonment in a body you don't like. Food evolves from your jailer to your savior – offering you nothing less than you feeling good about yourself – inside and out.

Now it's time to make a shift. Let's quit eating and get moving. In fact, let's wiggle our butts right into those pants with some exercise!

WHAT YOU NOW KNOW...

- Drinking milk and eating dairy products is a choice, not a necessity.

- Fresh, whole fruits and vegetables provide all the calcium we need.

- Cheese is addictive.

- Dairy products cause "little" problems: headaches, earaches, stomachaches, sniffing, sinusitis, congestion, colds, bronchitis, eczema, PMS, mood swings.

- Dairy products are linked to big problems: cancer, heart disease, stroke, diabetes, hypertension, Parkinson's, Crohn's, ulcerative colitis, irritable bower syndrome, multiple sclerosis, lupus, atherosclerosis, and rheumatoid arthritis.

- In this country, osteoporosis is not caused by the lack of calcium. It is caused by what you eat that leaches the calcium out of your bones.

- Look to nature for commonsense answers: where do cows get their calcium to grow big bones and produce milk? Certainly not milk.

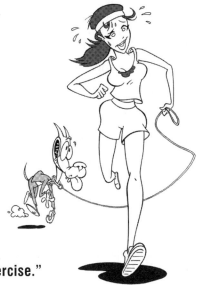

Chapter 15

Panting in Your Pants

"Yeah, but I hate to exercise."

- The "Do Something" Principle
- Your Great Big Buts

Confusion about weight loss and food is understandable. It *is* confusing! That's precisely why this book focuses on helping you learn to make more, better food choices and to incorporate a practical, step-by-step strategy into your daily life so that you can shed that fat – for life, not just for the sprint of a few months.

However, as confusing as food is, there's absolutely no confusion about exercise. To step into your pants, you must move your body! You already know that, and you certainly don't need me to tell you. So? Why aren't you?

Sure, reducing your calorie intake by adding and filling up on nature's best – fresh, whole fruits and vegetables – will get you into those pants. But who wants to jiggle with that hard-earned, sexy wiggle? You're doing yourself and your bottom side a huge disservice if you choose (yes, it's a choice!) to neglect the critical calorie expenditure part of the weight loss equation – fitness.

I will not belabor the point. It's simple. If you want your body to look, feel, and work its best, then you must exercise. Lots of experts and books can help you get started. You can even hire a personal trainer to give you a jumpstart. But, really, don't make this complicated. We're talking about putting on a pair of sneakers and going for a walk. How complicated is that?

THE "DO SOMETHING" PRINCIPLE

"But, but, but….I hate to exercise!"

I'm sure you have lots of excuses for not exercising. Perhaps you hate it, or you love it but don't have enough time or energy. Whatever it is, if you're not in the habit of exercising for one hour a day, every day, I suggest you try the "Do Something" Principle. This principle, taught to me by one of my mentors, Jeff Smith, can be applied to every aspect of life, including exercise.

Let's be very realistic. It's highly unlikely that you'll hop from no or sporadic exercising to a full sixty-minute-a-day program. So before you go into overload and give up before you even begin, forget the ideal and get real – just "do something." Start with baby steps. Those baby steps lead to gigantic leaps.

Even if you start by taking a walk for fifteen minutes, it's a whole lot better than sitting on the couch and eating chocolate. Look for spots in your day to squeeze in a bit of exercise. If you have ten minutes of down time before dinner, instead of watching TV, why not slip into those sneaks and go for a quick walk? If you get up too late to go to the gym for a full workout, instead of skipping exercise altogether, do some sit-ups or push-ups, or just stretch on your bedroom floor. If you've been working at your computer for hours, take a well-needed, short break and do a few yoga poses or squats. Consider making good use of your TV time. Instead of sitting, walk on a treadmill or use free weights to exercise your arms, shoulders, and chest while watching your squawk box.

And, remember to do the obvious little things that can add up to big calories burned over time, if you do them regularly. Park farther away from the store. Use the stairs instead of the elevator. Ride your bike to work. Play outside with your children or grandchildren. Get out of your chair as often as possible at work or at home. Grow some beautiful flowers or fresh fruits and veggies in your garden and get some exercise besides. Go for a walk with a friend instead of going to lunch or dinner. (Why do we always have to eat when we socialize?). Think outside the food box and inside the exercise box. With a bit of awareness and imagination, you'd be surprised at how effortless it can be to exercise more, and in ways that will also enrich your life.

The Next Step – A Regular Exercise Routine

When you're ready to incorporate a consistent, exercise program into your day, ask yourself a few questions to help you put exercise on auto-pilot – as normal an every day activity as sleeping and eating fruits and vegetables. This will help keep your exercise routine doable for you.

1. **What kind of exercise is right for me?**

   Do the exercise you like the best (or hate the least). If it's walking, perfect. Stick with it. That preference could change along the way, but then again, maybe not. If you're doing only one kind of exercise, make sure you're doing something cardiovascular (usually aerobic), which strengthens your most important muscle – your heart. Walking, hiking, biking, and swimming are great cardiovascular exercises. Or, perhaps you'd enjoy learning how to kayak, snowshoe, or cross-country ski. If physical problems preclude you from one physical activity, do another. For example, if you have knee problems, swim or row on a machine – low-impact activities. If you have shoulder problems, try biking or stepping on the elliptical machine. If you're breathing and can move, you can exercise. Whatever it is, find something you already like doing, or at least think you could like.

2. **How many days of the week will I exercise?**

If you want to jump right into working out seven days a week, more power to you. That's great. However, if seven days a week sounds too overwhelming for you at this point, start out building your routine exercise program by exercising four days a week, taking weekends off, and any weekday you choose. Try it for twenty minutes at a time, and give yourself a big atta-girl (or atta-guy) every time you finish. You're following the "Do Something" Principle, and that's what counts. Later on, you may want to alter the kind of exercise you do on different days, as in walking one day and doing yoga the next, or doing both on the same day, but then again, maybe not. Take it one day at a time and don't even think about other possibilities until you're naturally ready.

3. **What time investment am I looking at?**

As we said, sixty minutes a day is ideal, but if you're just starting or you're unable and/or unwilling to exercise a full hour, no worries – just do something and gradually build up. Push yourself. Think of those pants. I'll never forget what my little brother told me when we were kids growing up in the country, "Les, you can always do more than you think you can." And he was right, on many levels. His words have carried me through many a workout, physical and otherwise.

4. **What time of day works best for me?**

Whatever works with your schedule and natural energy levels is the best time of day for you. However, watch out for your old habits. If you always "plan to exercise after work" and something always comes up, choose a better time of day.

Personally, I prefer to exercise first thing in the morning (as in 5:45 am). Not only do I get it over and done with, but it wakes me up and primes my body and mind for the day. Even if you don't think you're a morning person, you may want to try it. You'd be surprised how quickly exercise can perk you up, and without the black brew.

5. **Where will I exercise?**

Each of us is different. Do you enjoy a favorite place to walk? Do you like to exercise at home using your own aerobic exercise machine, doing calisthenics, or lifting weights? Do you stay more on track if you join a gym, forming work-out relationships with other people who hold you accountable? Whatever works for you, do it!

6. Who or what can make exercise more fun and even educational?

If a partner helps keep you in the exercise groove, then find one. Don't give up until you do. It's amazing how quickly the time flies when you walk and chat as opposed to walking by yourself. Not only that, if you have a commitment to meet someone, you'll get there – no matter what excuse pops up. If you prefer to exercise alone, then of course a partner is a non-issue.

Music, television, educational and motivational CDs, or books-on-tape can transform exercise from boring into well-spent, pleasurable time. Again, figure out what works the best for you to keep you on track.

7. What sneakers should I wear?

This sounds like a no-brainer, but many people don't wear the right footwear for exercise and even in everyday life. Your footwear is very important to support your feet, your spine, and the rest of your structure. Invest in excellent sneakers - this is not the time to be cheap. Get excellent arch support, a roll bar, and motion control. In fact, use those three exact terms when scoping out sneakers for yourself. Most brands of sneakers market a wide-ranged assortment, but most don't come with those three things. In general, the higher the numbers on the sneakers and the more expensive, the better-made and the more supportive they are. You get what you pay for. Expect to spend at least $100 a pair and replace them as soon as they wear down. And most important of all, make sure they fit you properly.

8. **How can I stop myself from getting discouraged?**

As with building better food habits, be patient and kind to yourself. With time, excuses slip away and daily exercise becomes more automatic, even fun. You will get off track countless times. So what? Don't waste your energy by wallowing in guilt and "shoulda, woulda, couldas." Once again, the only slip up is to give up. Just get back on track again using the "Do Something" Principle.

YOUR GREAT BIG BUTS

Speaking of excuses, which "yeah, but" is going to stop you from moving that body today? Go ahead, if you're bold enough, confess. And as you're sounding off, listen to your own big buts and giggle – at yourself.

"But, but, but…no matter how much I exercise, I can't lose weight – what's the point?"

I hear this question all the time, and my answer is always the same: "Unless you're a high-performance athlete, it's almost impossible to lose significant weight by just exercise alone. If you're eating too many calories, exercise won't stop those calories from turning into the fat you wear. For example, you must walk eleven miles *at one time* to lose just one pound of fat. How can you possibly "burn off" those excess calories you try to rationalize away with exercise? Burning off calories is much harder than skipping calories from the get-go. No question about it – the best way to lose weight is by filling up on calorie-low, nutrient-rich fruits and vegetables. And then, the exercise provides bonus weight loss, shaving off even more calories, and thereby promoting quicker weight loss and better health."

"But, but, but...I don't have time."

I knew you were going to say that, even though both you and I know better! After accounting for the basics – eating, sleeping, working, commuting – according to Dr. John McDougall, M.D., in *The McDougall Program: 12 Days to Dynamic Health*, the average person has 69 hours in the rest of his or her week. So, what are you doing with all your extra hours? Even if you steal 7 of those hours to move your body, you still have 62 hours left to chat online, talk on the phone, watch TV, and go shopping.

The question isn't, "Do you have time?" The question is "Do you have your priorities straight?" Your body must come first; everything else comes second.

"But, but, but...exercise is so inconvenient."

Can't exercise because the list of life gets in the way? Think differently! Exercise gives you the convenience and thrill of feeling good, sustaining high energy, getting your body in shape, preventing diseases, and feeling good about you.

"But, but, but...I'm too tired."

Three things give you energy: carbohydrates from unrefined fruits and vegetables, adequate sleep, and getting oxygen to your brain and all of your cells. How do you supercharge your body with oxygen? Exercise! Too tired to exercise? Make yourself do it anyway. In the end, it will feed your energy reserves, not deplete them.

"But, but, but...my husband won't walk with me."

You're a big girl. Go by yourself or find another walking partner. It no longer serves you to blame your husband or anyone else for your choices. If you want to do it, you will. If you really want a walking buddy, find one. But please walk by your lonesome until you do.

"But, but, but...I have no place to exercise."

I suggest you open your eyes and look again. If you have to, you can put a stationary treadmill or bicycle in the smallest room in your home, and you'd still probably have space for a small TV for entertainment while you sweat. It may not be your first choice, but if you understand how important exercise is, then you'll make do. And I suspect your options are not quite this limited. Most of us have access to some sort of street, sidewalk, park, or live within a reasonable distance of a gym.

"But, but, but...I don't want to over do."

It's always important to start slowly and condition your body so you don't injure yourself. Make sure you take the time to warm up and cool down each time you work out. If you begin a new weight lifting program, expect to be sore for the first few weeks. Use common sense and listen to what your body tells you. If you're really worried, or if you have any health issues or physical limitations that concern you, make sure you talk to your health practitioner before starting any new program.

"But, but, but...I exercise enough at work or at home."

Physical work as part of your normal day is a great way to move your body. However, it doesn't burn the same amount of calories or cause the same benefits to your body as a good, "glowing" exercise session that keeps your heart rate elevated. Unless you really get your heart rate up and keep it there for at least forty minutes as part of your work or home routine, you probably aren't getting your daily quota.

"But, but, but…it's too cold."

…Or too hot…or too dark…or too sunny…or too windy…or look – it could rain – there's a wisp of a cloud.

Pick an excuse, any excuse, and keep picking excuses until you excuse yourself right out of the ability to exercise and directly into the grave. Having trouble making the choice to walk? Think how much trouble it would be to lose the option to walk, due to a major stroke or the loss of your legs from diabetes.

"But, but, but…I'm too lazy."

There you go – shedding denial and donning honesty. I applaud you. Awareness is always the first step to raising yourself to the next level. However, perhaps you're not lazy at all. Perhaps you really don't get the exercise-pants-health connection so exercise stays at the bottom of your list. After all, look at what you've done in your lifetime that took a tremendous amount of discipline and hard work – school, babies, teenagers (and living to tell the tale), marriage, single parenting, home projects, your career, yard cleaning, taking care of grandkids or aging parents. You are not lazy – you've done at least some of those things, all of which are much harder and more time consuming than walking for an hour.

"But, but, but…it's been over 21 days of exercise, and I'm still fighting with it."

Twenty-one days to form a habit? Yeah, right. Try twenty-one years! Whoever made up that adage had to be delusional! Without exaggeration, it took me twenty-five years to wake up in the morning and go exercise, without getting beat up in the "I will"/"I won't" war. I will exercise-I won't exercise. I will exercise-I won't exercise. And I like to exercise! How long will the battle go on for that unfortunate person who hates to exercise? Certainly longer than 3 weeks!

"It's all about baby steps…getting up…and panting."

My point here is this: whatever your excuses are, it's important to get past them to look and feel the way you want. The key to life, after all, is movement. The opposite of movement is death. The sooner you get connected in to how important exercise is to the number and quality of your days, the more you'll have the burning desire to stay in the exercise groove, right along with eating the 10+10 way.

Check out the conclusion of this astounding 8-year, 32,000 people study at the Cooper Institute for Aerobics: Inactive individuals are more likely to die prematurely than people who have all three major risk factors for early death – high cholesterol, high blood pressure *and* smoking combined, *if* the people with those risk factors exercise daily. Did you get that? If you have all three risk factors but you exercise daily, your chances of living longer are greater than the person who has none of these risk factors but doesn't exercise regularly.

So deafen your mind to sabotaging self-talk, lace up those good sneakers, put one foot in front of the other, get up after every fall, and baby step your way to a daily exercise program. And then, take a moment to revel in the wonderment of you and all that you're capable of.

As Jim Rohn, business philosopher says, the pain of regret weighs tons while the pain of discipline weighs ounces. Rewards, way beyond imagination and shedding fat, will be yours if you make the effort to pant in your pants today and every day, for the rest of your days.

WHAT YOU NOW KNOW...

- To add years to your life and life to your years, you've got to move.

- Just "Do Something" every day.

- Your own big buts that keep you from firming up that jiggle in those pants.

- Exercise doesn't take time, it gives you time when it counts – at the end of your life.

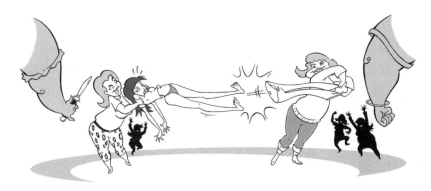

Chapter 16

Seven Sneaky Sisters Stealing Your Pants

Beware of the Seven Sneaky Sisters

- Wendy Whiner

- Frieda Fear

- Patty Perfect

- Betty Bored

- Annie Antsy

- Dena Denial

- Greta Greedy

So...picture yourself in six months.

You've lost fifteen pounds of fat. You're cruising full speed ahead in the 10+10 groove. You're excited. In fact, you're unstoppable. Those pants power your forward momentum. The longer you eat the 10+10 way, the more sense it makes, and the easier it gets. And you like it. You love feeling full and satisfied, without the guilt and fear of slipping up. In fact, you're wondering why you hadn't thought of eating like this before. You can't imagine ever going back to your old ways, especially since your pants are getting baggier by the week! No doubt about it – you're feeling good!

And then...

They're Baa-aack!

Just when you're feeling comfortable, invincible even, one or more of the seven sneaky sisters, uninvited and unexpected, crashes your private party. These sisters are our own, self-created personalities – the ones that rear their ugly heads and try to dominate and control you. Their mission: to sabotage your weight loss and body best success and you're feeling good about you.

Let's introduce them: Wendy Whiner, Frieda Fear, Patty Perfect, Betty Bored, Annie Antsy, Dena Denial, and Greta Greedy. Sometimes they work alone, playing you like a cat plays with a cornered mouse – toying, teasing, tormenting – before going in for the kill. Sometimes they team up and attack from all directions, overwhelming you and creating chaos, confusion, and frustration.

They use different tactics. But in the end they invade your mind, and the results are the same: you give up, feeling like a hopeless failure one more time.

Let's line up the sisters and see if you recognize them.

Wendy Whiner

Wendy Whiner is the easiest sister to spot, or rather, to hear. Her distinctive voice gives her away – an incessant, grating, high-pitched whine that loves to complain. "I hate to chew so much." "I can't find enough fruit this time of year." "The apples aren't crisp enough." "The Romaine lettuce is so expensive."

My suggestion: when you hear that twang coming, don't walk, run in the opposite direction. If you can't lose her, insert pointer fingers in ears, hum a little tune, and jump up and down. Do whatever you can to shut her out. After doing so well with 10+10, you don't want your mind to get infected by Wendy Whiner's whines.

Frieda Fear

And then there's Frieda Fear, much quieter than Wendy Whiner. She sneaks up without your even knowing it and hits with full force, paralyzing you. Her weapon: fear. Fear of upsetting a spouse, fear of not being liked by your children, fear of offending a friend, fear of insulting a dinner hostess, fear of making a guest uncomfortable, and fear of making waves. Ultimately, fear of being a bother to someone else.

My suggestion: if Frieda Fear creeps into your mind, take a deep breath, look her in the eye, and walk right past her. Do what you know is right for you. In the end, if you're better off, everyone else will be better off.

Penny Perfect

You know Penny Perfect. She thinks that she's a notch or two above us mere mortals. She doesn't *think* she's perfect, she *is* perfect – at least in the world according to Penny Perfect. The problem is, she makes you want to be just like her – perfect.

I hate to be the one to shatter delusion, but no matter what Miss Penny has to say, you're not perfect and will never be perfect. And guess what? You don't need to be perfect (whew) for the 10+10 program to work for you – not even close. If you hold yourself up to the standards of Penny Perfect, the first time you stray from your original good intentions and prepared plan (and you will), frustration will flair and disappointment will dominate. You'll beat yourself up for messing up, proving to yourself that this plan just doesn't work, or that it works, but you're a failure.

But you didn't fail – you're just not Penny Perfect. Getting off track is another opportunity for awareness, growth, and proving to yourself that you've got what it takes to get back on track again and again.

My suggestion: The next time Miss Goody Too-Big-For-Her-Britches comes around, give her a boot right in those britches by taking a deep breath and being patient with yourself. Nobody's perfect. Don't hold yourself up to unrealistic expectations or you'll fail. Expect a lot of yourself, but not perfection.

Betty Bored

Betty Bored is spoiled and loves to spoil you too, just to make her feel better about her own bad habits. Watch out for her. She's a master seductress, ruled by her taste buds that crave certain flavors and tastes. When her taste buds are happy, Betty Bored is happy. When her buds cry "boring," Betty Bored gets, well, bored. She gets bored by all the good foods – fruits, salads, and vegetables, no matter how much variety. Yet, she never gets bored by the bad stuff, no matter how often she indulges in the same thing.

With a little time and persistence, your taste buds will get used to the best-for-you foods, and you'll actually start enjoying them – craving them even. But just between you and me, Betty Bored seems quite content to stay enslaved to those little buds, just the way they are. She likes her prison. She's used to it. Be cautious of her sweet talk and wily ways that lure you in. Her prison can be your prison.

My suggestion: Ignore Betty Bored's narrow mindset. You're going to get into those pants, by golly. Show those taste bud brats of yours who's boss. Sure, they'll holler and whine, but who cares? The rest of your body will thank you. And, eventually, those little guys will come around and learn to love the flavors created to keep you alive and kickin' up your heels in those pants.

Annie Antsy

When Annie Antsy wants something, she wants it right now. Like losing weight. And if she doesn't lose it fast enough, she gives up – just like that. I'm so sorry, Ms. Annie. It just doesn't work like that. It took years to build up that fat, and it takes time to get it off and keep it off.

Sure, you may be able to drop weight more quickly by starving and depriving yourself. But the minute your hunger drive takes over – and it will – or you just get sick of all the "can't haves," and rebel, the fat comes back to its favorite hang-outs.

Annie Antsy may be fun to hang out with, for a while, but fun quickly turns into impatience and discontent with perfectly reasonable forward progress in a reasonable time – like 2.5 pounds a month, 30 pounds in a year, and the grand total of 60 pounds in two years. Impatience and discontent lead to giving up, for the 20th or 50th or 500th time.

My suggestion: Smile sweetly at Annie Antsy, wave, and move on. Adopt Patty Patience as your new best friend.

Dena Denial

Dena Denial is like a snorting, blind bull, stomping her hoof in the sand, ready to charge. She's the sister who's layered with rolls, looks and feels crummy, but still knows it all. She knows her way is the only way with no room for improvement. Not only that, she knows what's best for you, too, and doesn't hesitate to impart her wisdom. And Dena Denial can come from more places than just your own head. She could be a mother, a sister, friend, neighbor, teacher, doctor, pastor, author, talk-show host, reporter, or even a weight-loss and health expert.

My suggestion: when a bull comes charging at you, step out of the way. Don't explain. Don't argue. In fact, don't talk – at least not about food and you. There's no point. She'll either refuse to budge, or she'll charge. Either way, she'll leave you shaken and confused. Make a mad dash out of her pen as quickly as possible. Stick with what you know is right. It's not your job to prove it to anyone else. That's my job.

Greta Greedy

Nothing's good enough for Greta Greedy. Perhaps you've met her and know what I mean.

Greta Greedy decides on the doable weight loss goal of 2.5 pounds a month, even though it sounds low to her. One month later her weight has dropped 7.5 pounds. Is her response elation, giddiness, and a bubbly bounce? Not at all. It's, "I could've done better had I only done such and such." Doesn't matter that she lost three times her goal. Nope, still wasn't good enough for Greta Greedy. Next month – more of the same. Greta loses more than her goal, but no, still isn't good enough. She woulda, shoulda, coulda lost more. She's disappointed again – even though she's met her goals and beyond. And so the pattern goes. No matter how successful she is, no matter how much weight she loses, Greta is never satisfied. She's always greedy for more, and more is never enough.

Then the inevitable happens. Greta Greedy gives up because she can never fulfill her self-created, impossible expectations.

My suggestion: it won't be easy, but detach yourself from Greta Greedy. Once she latches on, you'll continually feel "not good enough," no matter how well you're doing. Start out by knowing that you *are* good enough and hang on to that. Keep your clear intentions and well-defined goals in the forefront of your mind. Then track all of the specific changes and action steps you take every day in every month to reach those goals. They add up in a hurry. Feel good about each and every one of them, as well as your commitment and effort to be the all-time champ in this weight war.

And for goodness sakes, congratulate yourself every step of the way. It's not easy to lose weight and keep it off over the long haul, especially with Greedy and her sisters vying for your pants. Any amount you lose is a victory and worthy of a proud stance, a feel-good smile, and at least one satisfied, backward glance in the mirror, followed by a great big, "Yes!"

You've got your eye on them...

So, now I've done my job and warned you. It's your job to take heed. These mindsets happen to all of us – even me. We get caught up in the whirlwind and thrill of a new program. Then, over time, the flame can dim as self-doubt, insecurities, fears, and the love of old habits creep in, stealing those pants away. This time, keep those pants in plain sight at all times, and they'll be yours!

WHAT YOU NOW KNOW...

- The biggest block between you and those pants: YOU!

- Make the commitment, hunker down, and follow through with that do it or die determination – no matter which sisters come knocking on your door.

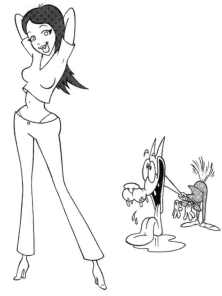

Chapter 17

The First Step into Your Pants

"How do I get started?"

- Your New-You Plan of Action

- How to Shop

- Suggestions for Organizing your Kitchen

- A Guide to Your First Week of Meals

- Building Your Dream House

Now you've got all the know-how about 10+10. But do you really know how to start? How do you take that first step to the rest of your life?

This last chapter is all about helping you turn your newfound knowledge into a step-by-step plan for action. I will help you shop, reorganize your kitchen, and teach you how to plan week-at-a-glance meals, all important steps to make your transition to 10+10 as smooth and effortless as possible.

YOUR NEW-YOU PLAN OF ACTION

Remember the "Do Something Principle" from Chapter 15? You can apply it to food choices as well as exercise. The most important thing is that you "do something." It's kind of like getting into a pool. You may be the type of person who prefers to take things very slowly by dipping your toe in and testing. In terms of 10+10, for instance, you may choose to eat just fruit in the morning before venturing into any other meals. That's a pretty easy, enjoyable transition for most. Or, you may be the type who stands on the edge, takes a deep breath, and jumps right in. Of course, the faster you immerse yourself in 10+10, the faster you'll see results. But don't fret, you toe-dippers, slow and steady works, too – it just takes more time and patience right along with it.

Whether you are a toe-dipper or a full-body plunger or somewhere in between, if you have the want and the will, by following the 10+10 way, you'll get there – at your own pace. Of the utmost importance, however, is that you design a clear plan of specific actions tailored to you, *your* vision, *your* wants, *your* needs, and *your* daily life. And then, after you plan, you can start the forward momentum by following your plan and sticking to it.

If, per chance, that plan needs to be tweaked or even changed completely later down the road, then you can adjust it accordingly, as long as you still follow the 10+10 principles. This initial plan is merely the springboard into your new way of eating. It will change and develop as you change and grow. Fully embrace what works for you, and discard what clearly doesn't. Be aware and honest with yourself. Be open. And get ready to be flexible with yourself. Change when *you* need a change. Push yourself when *you* need a push. Back off when *you* need a pressure release. After all, this is *your* plan.

Your plan of action

In my experience, the following steps are highly effective in creating and following an overall plan of action. If you sit down and focus, this planning process should take you no longer than half an hour.

1. **Formulate your one-year weight-loss goal.**

   This number should come from the assessment you took in Chapter 4. If, for any reason, you didn't complete that assessment or want to re-think your original number, here are some guidelines to help.

   First, think about whether or not your number is realistic for your lifestyle and your health. Being honest with yourself is vital to your success. This number may not be your overall fit-into-those pants number. Remember, take it one feel-good pound at a time. This is only your first year. There are other years for those other pounds.

   I strongly recommend that you consider a **30-pound weight loss goal for this first year.** That is 2.5 pounds a month. Less than a pound a week. If you are a person who is going to tip toe into 10+10 really, really slowly (which is completely fine!), be prepared for your weight loss to be a little less than this.

   A lot of people tell me this seems slow. Remember, this is not a magical quick-fix. This is good old-fashioned commitment and hard work. When this first year flies by and you reach your weight loss goal, trust me, you will be thrilled with 30 pounds less of you looking back in the mirror! And then there's always the next twelve months to gradually take off more, if you need to, and that will thrill you beyond imagination. Patience is a huge virtue – especially when it comes to weight loss. After all, think about how long you have been building your weight up.

2. Write down your one-year weight-loss goal and say it out loud – every time you eat.

    It will say something like**: "I will lose _____ pounds by (date), exactly one year from today."** Put it in a very visible place so that you'll see it every day, like on the bathroom mirror, next to the scale, or even on the refrigerator door. And don't take it down until your year is over.

    Take it one step farther: tell one other person, just one, whom you *know* will support you and cheer you on. (Be sure this person is a cheerleader and not saboteur.) Report your progress to her (or him) consistently every month. Being held accountable is a huge kingpin to losing those pounds.

    Along with your weight-loss goal, I'd also like you to write down at least five, and up to ten, other yearlong goals that are important to you. Make sure they are very real and relevant to you. Keep them close by and look at them several times a week.

    Examples of these goals are: safely cut down or eliminate specific medications (write down which ones), lower my blood pressure, cholesterol, and/or triglycerides, get my blood glucose under 100 consistently so I can safely get off diabetic medications (work with your doctor), exercise routinely, increase energy, feel better with fewer aches and pains, feel better about myself, and get into a size _____. Please keep in the forefront of your mind that if your weight-loss goal is met, most of these other goals will be met as well.

3. Write down your monthly weight-loss goal.

Break that 12-month, weight-loss goal into doable, bite-size chunks of one-month goals. For instance, the yearlong goal of 30 pounds can be broken down into the monthly goal of 2.5 pounds. And that certainly sounds doable, doesn't it?

Find a calendar that can be your personal calendar – no one else's – and write that 2.5 pounds on the top of every month, as in "March's weight-loss goal: 2.5 pounds."

4. Choose and write down five action steps.

So far so good? Good. This next step will take a little bit of time, but it will pay off in huge dividends. This is the "meat" (little joke there!) of your action plan: the specific action steps. Go back and skim Chapters 6, 7, and 8 – the breakfast, lunch, and dinner chapters. Pick out five, only five, key, practical ideas that sound the easiest for you to implement into your day right now, *starting today*.

On your calendar, write down these five action steps. If you are a toe-dipper, you may want to choose only one or two action steps to start off with. If you are a full-body plunger, pick out five, but *only* five. It's easy to get overexcited and bite off more than you can chew, which can cause you to get overwhelmed by it all and then choke and give up. Relax, this is a lifelong process. You can add different action steps every month if you'd like.

Here is an example of five common action steps.

1.) Eat only fruit throughout the morning.

2.) Eat daily a fill-me-up 10+10 salad for lunch.

3.) Eat dinner in order: salad, steamed vegetables, potato/ winter squash topped with avocado/tomato/guacamole or rice and/or bean dish. STOP eating when full. Eat meat/ fish/pasta last, if I must.

4.) Eat fruit, cut-up veggies, and raw, unsalted nuts and seeds for snacks.

5.) Walk 4 days a week for 30 minutes.

5. **Track your action steps and congratulate yourself.**

At the end of each day, write down the numbers that represent the specific action steps you completed on that day, right on the day in calendar.

For instance, if on Tuesday, April 1, 2008, you completed the first, second, fourth, and fifth action steps from your plan as I previously listed, simply write the number 1, 2, 4, and 5 on that day, April 1. This will help you:

1.) Stay on track to reach your yearlong goals.

2.) Keep a permanent record to refer back to when trying to figure out why you are or aren't losing as planned.

3.) Feel good about YOU. When you look back at an entire month, in a glance you can actually see the numbers of all action steps you completed. Then you can marvel at yourself and say with complete awe, "Look at *all* the things I did right." Your focus will shift from the negative – the couldas, shouldas, but didn'ts – to the positive.

Some women actually put little sticker smiley faces or stars on the calendar day every time they follow through with an action step. Oh, yes, we must always have fun! Just think, in one year's time you'll have a whole lot of smiley faces reflecting your one great, big smiley face. Atta-girl (or guy)! Be proud of you.

6. Weigh yourself monthly.

At the end of every month, weigh yourself and write it down by your month's weight goal on the specific month in your calendar. If you're on track with your monthly goal – great for you! If not, please don't fret, stew, guilt, or beat yourself up. Remember, you're in this for the long haul. One month is insignificant in the whole scheme of things.

Simply regroup. Get even more determined than ever. Look back at the action steps recorded on your calendar and see for yourself where you could improve and, even more significantly, where you are willing to improve. Modify your action steps the next month to better facilitate reaching your monthly weight-loss goal. Forgive me for nagging, but if you use your wiggle room too much, it will show on the scale. If you're serious about getting into those pants, then get serious about your monthly action steps. You can do this, one action step at a time!

7. Revisit action steps every month.

At the beginning of every month, look at your action steps from the previous month. Make any adjustments appropriate for you. If you decide to upgrade your exercise, then write down that new action step. If you'd rather just follow 10+10 for breakfast and lunch, not dinner just yet, then make sure your action steps show that change. Once an action step transforms into a habit that you know you will stick with, then drop it from your monthly action steps and replace it with another one. Those action steps, if you are fully engaged in your plan, will evolve as you evolve.

8. **Assess your year-end accomplishments.**

At the end of the year, look at your original, yearlong goals and all your monthly action steps. Assess where you started, how far you've come, and where you want to go from here. Remember, the measurement of your success is not just the number of pounds you lost but also the fulfillment of your other tangible goals and all those not-so-tangible goals, like feeling good about yourself and all those things you did *right* over the course of the year!

Formulate your new yearlong weight goal and 5-10 new health/lifestyle goals for the next year, as well as specific action steps for the next month, the first month of your new year. Remember, once an action step becomes automatic (as in you've done it every day for the past four months without thinking about it), you should replace it with a new or upgraded action step. This will keep you moving in a forward direction.

Now that you have a specific plan to follow, let's go shopping and put that plan into action. Let the 10+10 adventure begin!

HOW TO SHOP

When you go to the store next time, pretend it's a field trip and have fun. Explore the store, from the aisles and aisles of deplete-me foods to the feed-me foods tucked mostly in the fresh produce section. Notice all the different, fresh fruits and vegetables – some of which you grab every week and some of which you never knew existed.

If you are unfamiliar with a fruit, you could buy one and try it. If you have no idea how to pick one out, ask one of the grocers. You may be surprised and delighted by the treat of a whole new array of flavors and textures. If you are unfamiliar with a vegetable, you could find out what it is and how to best prepare it by asking someone or searching through cookbooks or the Internet.

However, after opening your eyes to all the possibilities available to you, I suggest that the bulk of what you buy, especially at first, consists of familiar fruits and vegetables – just to make it easier for you. Diving headfirst into new foods and new recipes can be tremendously time consuming and overwhelming.

The simpler the better.

The simpler you eat, the better it is for you. In other words, what can be easier, and better for you, than eating a whole apple (several of them), munching a whole carrot, or filling up on a large, 10+10 fresh, vegetable salad with all those vegetables that you already know so well? For dinner, throw in those more filling, very familiar potatoes, sweet potatoes, yams, winter squashes, brown rice, and beans, and you'll be full and very satisfied. And the best part, they are extraordinarily easy to make and cheap to buy.

So start simple, follow though with simple, and end simple. Then, if you are so inclined, gradually build your repertoire of fresh fruits, vegetables, new recipes, and new dishes. Or, if you're satisfied with the fresh fruits and veggies you already know, stick with them.

Warning ladies! We love to make more work for ourselves than necessary and then complain about it. As I mentioned previously, I don't know about you but I'm tired of spending my life in the kitchen. There's a great, big, beautiful playground out there, called the world, for us to enjoy.

Do not make food shopping and meal planning and preparation more complicated than needed. 10+10 is simple. Please do yourself the huge favor of learning how to enjoy simple foods and simple meals. Your body will thank you. Your family may grumble a bit here and there with the changes, but they can still enjoy their old foods while you follow the 10+10 plan of adding and filling up on the best-for-you foods first and then wiggling (if you must!) with your family.

Fill up your cart in the same order you eat - with feed-me foods first!

Just like filling up your body with the 10+10 feed-me foods first, fill up your cart with the feed-me foods first, enough to last several days. Start with the fruit. Move on to vegetables. Then go through your weekly dinners. Spend most of your time and money in the fresh produce section and then in the whole grains and beans section if those need replenishing. (You should keep a large store of different grains and beans at home, so you won't need to shop for these every week.) Just like when you're eating, fill up your cart with 80% feed-me foods. Then, after getting all the good-for-you stuff, if you must, venture into the aisles of deplete-me foods and grab your 20%, along with anything your family wants.

I have found that shopping twice a week is plenty. Shop one time for some longer-keeping fruits and vegetables (it make take you a few months to figure out exactly how long certain fruits and veggies keep), whole grains, beans, dry goods, and any extra items you need for your family and your own wiggle room (if you must!). Go back a second time, later in the week, to restock fruits and vegetables. Lettuce, for example, along with spinach and other greens for salad, should be purchased a couple times a week. This second shopping trip will be a quick stop into the produce section and out. Shopping time: no more than 15 minutes.

It won't take long before the bulk of your food shopping can be done very efficiently in the produce section and without a list. Unless I have dry goods to pick up, I never use a list. I shop for the same basic fruits and vegetables and know the exact quantities I need.

It will take you a while to get 10+10 shopping down to a science. But, to start with, think about it this way: If you eat 10 servings of fruit for breakfast, you need 10 fruits a day times seven days. That's 70 servings of fruit. If you make two shopping trips, perhaps you'll buy three days worth (30 servings) the first time and four days worth (40 servings) the second time. Remember, larger fruits contain several servings and a carton of berries or a bunch of grapes contains several as well. The same goes for the salad portions.

As you get more familiar with your new eating habits, tweak what you buy to accommodate what you know you'll eat. The types of things you buy will vary with the seasons and availability. I get the fruits and veggies that appeal to me when I see them. Shopping the 10+10 way is really that simple.

Convenience Feed-me Fast Foods

Even though fresh fruits and vegetables are the fastest fast foods (open mouth, insert food, and chew), many supermarkets now carry even faster fast fruits and vegetables.

You'll find prepackaged, pre-washed lettuce, salad greens, spinach, cut and shredded vegetables from cabbage to broccoli, along with containers of cut-up, fresh fruits of all kinds. If you wash and cut up fruits and vegetables yourself, they are better for you and cheaper, but what the heck. These prepackaged fruits and vegetables are much better options than most other foods so if the convenience of it works for you, go for it.

However, be aware that some of the prepackaged vegetables may have things added to keep them fresh, or even have added sugar. For example, I recently discovered that some prepackaged, pre-washed spinach, labeled as "organic spinach," is washed in chlorine and gassed to keep it fresher longer. Like I said, beware of anything that has a label.

Now that you have a shopping cart full of 10+10 feed-me foods, what do you do with all that produce once you get it back home? It's time to purge and reorganize your kitchen.

SUGGESTIONS FOR ORGANIZING YOUR KITCHEN

Take an objective survey of your kitchen. Start with the pantry. Yikes! Scary. How many canned, packaged, bagged, and boxed depleting foods do you have in there? Probably a lot, am I right? What do you say we clean out the old and make way for the new? As far as that idea of being wasteful, let it go. These are the foods that are keeping you trapped. Get rid of them. Throw out the already-opened foods and donate unopened foods to your local food bank. If there are items that your family eats and won't get rid of, designate one shelf to those items and restrict them to that shelf. I would recommend relegating them to the very bottom shelf as a direct reflection of their unwelcome status. Keep them out of your sight as much as possible.

For you toe-dippers out there, relax! Sort and discard at your own pace, but definitely start by getting rid of all those depleting foods that you know you're not going to eat. Keep anything that you're not quite sure about (or you could get a bit daring as you go, take a deep breath, and throw it away). This cleaning does not have to be a one-time event. It's a process. Again, "do something" to get the forward momentum going.

For all you full-body plungers, take that flying leap and dive right in! Get a few large boxes and some garbage bags and say good riddance to all those foods that go directly from your lips to your hips! You're done with them forever, and you don't need them hanging around trying to lure you back in. Trust yourself, but don't tempt yourself.

Hang on to the canned kidney beans, canned vegetables, whole grains, dried beans, and even whole-grain pastas. Check out the soups, sauces, and jarred juices to see how depleting they are. Decide whether they make the cut or not. With most foods, have a party tossing out the canned and packaged foods that you know you never want to eat again, like oils, Jell-o, cake mixes, macaroni and cheese, Ramen, cereals, microwave popcorn, and all the rest of the bad-guys you've been collecting for years.

This purging process is exhilarating, liberating even. Cleaning out your cupboards is the direct reflection of cleaning out old ideas and habits that no longer serve you and creating the space for new ideas to emerge and grow into healthy habits.

Your Fridge

Your refrigerator is next. Watch out! You never know what will jump out at you when you open that door. Your mission is to search and destroy. Out with the bad, including those condiments and oily salad dressings on the door, and in with the good! You want as much space as possible for your 10+10 variety of fresh fruits and vegetables.

Your crisper drawers are perfect for keeping the green-leafy lettuces, spinach, and celery as fresh as possible (make sure you bag them up before putting them in the crispers). The newly cleaned off shelves are ideal for storing and organizing your fruits and other vegetables. Yes, that's right – you can let your fruits and veggies out of the drawers. They get shelf space now! I store like fruits together, unbagged, on one or two shelves. I pull the older fruits to the front and put the newly purchased ones toward the back. I keep the vegetables in the clear, plastic bags I buy them in and place them together on a shelf as well. I always have one bag with all the vegetables (except the lettuce) I need immediately for a salad, so they're very accessible.

Because I have no condiments or salad dressings on the door shelves, I use those shelves for the avocados, lemons, and limes I use in salads, as well as vegetables I use in salads every day, like cucumbers, red peppers, and onions.

Your Counter

Place the fruits that don't need to be refrigerated in nice bowls or on plates on your counter. Also, some fruits need to ripen. Once they're ripe, I either eat them, or, if too many ripen at the same time, they go into the refrigerator. Keep your counter fully stocked with fruits so they're in plain sight as all times, and you can grab them quickly. Most fruits taste best at room temperature. So, leaving out your supply for the next morning helps a lot. Then, when you're hungry, grab what's right in front of you – fruit! If you are at work, you can keep a fruit bowl on your desk, or pack your meals in reusable to-go containers, like Tupperware. I check the status of the fruit every day to figure out which ones to eat, which ones to move to the refrigerator, which ones to keep on the counter, and which ones I need to buy. Avocados, for instance, are lined up in a row, and, as they ripen, they go into the refrigerator. I eat the refrigerated avocados first.

As you get used to the larger quantities of fresh fruits and vegetables, you will discover for yourself the most efficient way to organize and reorganize your kitchen until it becomes a fine-tuned, weight-loss machine with all the booby traps cleared out!

"Must have" tools

Make sure you have the right tools. They really save time and frustration. These are all the basic tools you need for 10+10. If you don't have them all, start collecting. They will make life a lot easier:

- Large salad spinner – 10¼" in diameter (Note: the bottom should be solid – no holes)

- Large cutting board – 20¾" x 15"

- Chef's knife (sharp) with 8" blade, wider at handle

- Boning knife (sharp) with straight, narrow 6" blade

- Peeler, julienner

- Large bowl for salad

- Two oversized spoons or fork and spoon for tossing salad

- Vegetable steamer basket – stainless steel

- Rice/grain cooker

- Good blender/chopper to puree and chop (I love my Cuisinart)

- Large stainless steel pot to cook beans and soups

- Medium stainless steel pot to steam vegetables

- Stainless steel wok or pan to sauté (in water) vegetables (don't use Teflon or coated cookware)

- Juicer (on your wish list) – contact me for recommendations – I'm an old-time juicer of almost thirty years

A GUIDE TO YOUR FIRST WEEK OF MEALS

The following week of meals will give you an idea of how to think about planning a 10+10 week of food. Some of the fruits are seasonal so make substitutes with available fruits. Some fruits I buy every week all year round, like bananas, apples, oranges, grapefruits, and grapes. Some people find that planning a week like this and making a detailed shopping list helps them. In my experience, this eating method is so simple that I don't need to take the time to do that. But, by all means, do what you know will work for you.

Note: Remember, breakfast fruits are eaten throughout the morning. Also, all salads can be dressed with balsamic vinegar and lemon juice or your favorite oil-free, dairy-free, additive-free, sugar-free salad dressing. As for the 10+10 salads, don't measure and count your vegetables. The amounts I have included in Monday and Tuesday's salad portions are suggestions to get you started. Add more or less as you like.

Substitute where you need. Absolutely any fruit or vegetable herein can be substituted for any other fruit or vegetable.

Monday	Tuesday
· Breakfast – ¼ honeydew melon, 2 bananas, 2 oranges, 1 grapefruit, 2 apples, ½ cup of fresh raspberries.	· Breakfast – ¼ pineapple, 2 apples, 4 small to medium plums, 1 nectarine, 2 peaches.
· Lunch – Large 10+10 veggie salad with the following: several handfuls of chopped Romaine lettuce, spinach, and arugula; ¼ sliced red onion, ½ avocado, a handful of shaved carrot slices (use a vegetable peeler to shave the carrots), ⅓ cucumber, 8-12 cherry tomatoes, 1 diced red bell pepper, a handful chopped raw broccoli. (Save a few large handfuls of the salad (undressed) for dinner. Eat the rest.) Follow the salad, if and only if you still want it, with a slice of whole wheat toast topped with avocado or a chopped tomato.	· Lunch – Large 10+10 salad with red leaf lettuce, spinach, ¼ red onion, a handful of baby carrots, steamed, diced potatoes left over from the night before (potatoes really help fill you up which is very important for weight loss and craving control), 1 green pepper, a handful raw cauliflower, 1 Roma tomato, ⅓ julienne zucchini, ⅓ chopped cucumber. If you're still hungry, eat some leftover asparagus from dinner or a handful of raw, unsalted, non-sugared pecans.
· Dinner – 1. Eat the remaining 10+10 salad from lunch (add more lettuce and veggies if you want a bigger salad). 2. Steamed green beans and asparagus. 3. Diced and steamed potato, topped with pureed avocado and/or fresh tomato salsa. (Steam 1 extra potato for your lunch salad tomorrow).	· Dinner – 1. Cut-up cucumbers, red peppers, carrot sticks, cauliflower with avocado or hummus dip. 2. Black bean and brown rice burritos with tomatoes, shredded lettuce, jalapeños, onions, guacamole wrapped in whole wheat tortilla shell.

Wednesday

· Breakfast –
½ honeydew, 2 kiwis, 2 mangos, 1 nectarine, 1 pear, 2 oranges, grapes.

· Lunch –
100% sprouted-grain sandwich with avocado, tomato, red pepper, onions, cucumber, and hummus spread (a nice change-up from salad), and a handful of raw, unsalted almonds.

· Dinner –
1. Make enough salad for dinner tonight, and for your lunch tomorrow, with Romaine and red leaf lettuce, arugula, carrots, cucumber, red pepper, zucchini, cauliflower, cherry tomatoes, green snap peas, sliced radishes, purple cabbage, and raw almonds. 2. Follow that with red lentil soup (see simple recipe). 3. If you are really hungry when you get to the soup, toast 1 slice of sprouted-grain bread to dip or steam a potato and pour the soup over the potato.

Thursday

· Breakfast –
Cooked whole oats with almond milk, blueberries, strawberries, raisins, apples, cinnamon, and a little raw honey (a reprieve from fruit only).

· Lunch –
Eat the salad you made at dinner last night. If you are still hungry, enjoy a warm bowl of leftover lentil soup.

· Dinner –
1. Again, make enough salad for dinner and lunch tomorrow, with Romaine, red leaf, arugula, 1 avocado, cherry tomatoes, cucumber, zucchini, broccoli, shaved fennel (from the bulb area), carrots, and raw, unsalted sunflower seeds. 2. Steamed broccoli and fennel (you can steam the bulb and the stems, after slicing it). 3. Black beans "stir-fried" in water with tomatoes, onion, chili powder, and cumin, topped with a little guacamole. (Save some beans for next day's salad – beans are very filling.)

Friday

· Breakfast –
2 bananas, 2 oranges, 2 apples, bunch of grapes, 1 mango, ¼ of your pineapple.

· Lunch –
Have the salad leftover from last night, along with some of your leftover bean/vegetable mixture.

· Dinner –
1. Make a salad with leftover lettuce and veggies and eat it while you cook, if you want to. 2. Steamed brown rice covered with a stir fry (in water or veggie broth) of broccoli, mushrooms, carrots, snap peas, zucchini, red onion, fresh ginger, and a bit of tamari sauce (like soy sauce). Top the veggies with finely chopped raw almonds and raw bean sprouts.

Saturday

· Breakfast –
¼ cantaloupe, 1 banana, 2 tangerines, 2 pears, grapes, the rest of your blueberries, strawberries, and raspberries or any other fruit you have left over.

· Lunch –
Make one large 10+10 salad to split between dinner and lunch with remaining lettuce, cucumber, carrots, Roma tomatoes, cherry tomatoes, broccoli, cauliflower, green and red peppers, and any other veggies lying around that look good to you. 2. If still hungry, make an open-faced, sprouted-grain sandwich with one slice of bread stacked with avocado, sprouts, lettuce, tomatoes, red peppers, and onions, spread with hummus.

· Dinner –
1. 10+10 salad leftover from lunch. 2. Spaghetti squash (excellent pasta substitute) topped with fresh tomato marinara sauce (see simple recipes).

Sunday

· Brunch with family –
This is wiggle time – sleep in
and then eat whatever you want.
You've earned it!

· Afternoon snacks –
1. raw nuts and seeds 2. any leftover fruit.

· Dinner –
1. 10+10 salad made of any leftover veggies 2. Grilled portobello
mushroom and yam topped with
avocado puree and fresh tomatoes.

Shopping List

Fruits

Apples	8
Avocado	6
Bananas	5
Cantaloupe	1
Honeydew	1
Oranges	6
Grapefruit	1
Kiwi	2
Mango	3
Nectarines	2
Pineapple	1 ripe
Plums	4
Peaches	2
Pears	3
Tangerines	2
Grapes	1 large bunch
Blueberries	1 fresh pint or frozen package
Strawberries	2 pints or frozen package
Raspberries	1 pint or frozen package

Vegetables

Romaine Lettuce	1 large head or bag
Red Leaf Lettuce	2 heads
Arugula	2 heads
Spinach	1 bunch or bag
Mushrooms	1 serving
Portobello	1
Red Onion	3 large
Yellow Onion	3 medium
Cherry Tomatoes	1 pint
Roma Tomatoes	6
Cucumber	3
Zucchini	1
Broccoli	1 head
Cauliflower	1 head

Red Peppers	3
Green Peppers	2
Green Snap Peas	2 handfuls
Green Beans	Large handful
Fennel	1 whole bulb
Carrots	3 lb bag
Radishes	2
White Potatoes	2
Yam/Sweet Potato	1
Asparagus	1 bunch
Jalapenos	4 (optional)
Bean Sprouts	1 package
Spaghetti Squash	1

Fresh Herbs/Spices

Cilantro	1 bunch
Basil	1 bunch
Fresh Ginger	1 small piece
Garlic	1 head

Grains/Beans

Red Lentils	1 bag
Whole Oats	1 container or a couple of pounds if bulk buying
Black Beans	1 bag, several pounds if bulk buying, or 1 can (if canned, no salt or oil, and preferably organic)
Brown Rice	1 container or a couple pounds if bulk buying (thoroughly wash all rice before steaming)

Breads

| 100% Sprouted-grain bread | 1 loaf (some brands, like Ezekiel, are sold in the freezer section) – store in the freezer and toast as needed |
| Whole wheat tortilla shells | 1 package – store in freezer and thaw as needed |

Other

Raw, unsalted almonds – 1 pound

Raw, unsalted sunflower seeds – ¼ pound

Salt-free or low sodium vegetable broth (preferably organic) – 1 box

Canned organic, salt-free, oil-free chopped tomatoes – 1

Hummus – 1 pre-made container or 2 batches of homemade hummus (see recipe below)

Cinnamon

Cumin

Chili Powder

Raw honey (unless you are 100% vegan)

Simple Recipes:

Avocado Spread/Guacamole – 1 avocado, squeeze of fresh lemon or lime juice, ½ diced tomato, ½ clove grated raw garlic (optional), handful of chopped cilantro – mash or puree together

Fresh Tomato Salsa – 1 cup diced tomatoes (any variety), ½ sliced red onion, 1 chopped jalapeno pepper (optional), a handful of chopped basil or cilantro (optional), a squeeze of lime juice

Hummus – 1 cup cooked/canned chick peas (garbanzo beans) in a food processor, along with ⅛ cup water, ¼ chopped white/yellow onion, and fresh herbs you like, a few cloves of grated garlic (optional), 2 tbsp Tahini (Note: Tahini is sesame paste. It is optional and can be found in grocery or health food stores), and a jalapeno (optional). Blend until a thick paste has formed. You can store hummus for a few weeks in the fridge.

Lentil Soup (feel free to substitute beans for lentils) – Cook 1 cup of red or green lentils in water or salt-free (or at least low-sodium) vegetable broth, as directed on the lentil package. Add an extra ½ cup of liquid. As the lentils are stewing, add some finely chopped yellow onion (about ½ cup), 1 finely chopped red pepper, 2 chopped/peeled tomatoes, 1 small chopped carrot, 1 chopped jalapeno (optional), 3-4 cloves of chopped garlic, a bay leaf, a teaspoon of cumin (or another spice you like), and some freshly ground black pepper. Add more liquid as the soup cooks if it gets too thick. After the lentils and vegetables are soft, take ½ cup of the soup and puree in a blender or food processor. Mix this back in with the soup. (This is a great tip to thicken any kind of soup and meld the flavors together.)

Fresh Tomato Marinara Sauce – In a sauce pan, combine 1 can salt-free, oil-free, organic chopped tomatoes, 1 chopped yellow onion, 2

tbsp finely chopped carrots, 4 cloves chopped garlic, a large handful of chopped basil, and some dried thyme (optional). Bring to a boil for 5 minutes and then reduce to a simmer for 35 minutes. You can usually keep this in the fridge for 7-10 days.

NOW YOU'VE GOT IT ALL

There you have it – all the tools you need to jump into 10+10 – a simple plan of action, shopping and organization tips, and a few meals to get you headed in the right direction. So? What are you waiting for? Now it's just a matter of putting on those sneakers and doing it! In no time at all, the effortful will magically transform into the effortless. And your body will have transformed, too.

BUILDING YOUR DREAM HOUSE

But before you run off to your 10+10 adventure, I must congratulate you for your interest, your diligence, and the deep-down guts it takes to step into the weight-loss arena one more time, for the last time. Your commitment to your body and health are an inspiration.

You've done a great job wading through all the nuggets of information, some of which you already knew, and some of which shocked the pants off you. I hope *Getting Into Your Pants* has left you well-informed and will continue to serve you well, opening one "ah-ha" door after another to raise your level of knowledge and awareness, allowing you to cut through the confusion and enabling you to use your own common sense as a guiding beacon of light.

Awareness and knowledge lead to self-evolvement and your vision of a new you with real goals and real hope. This vision, along with your clear intentions to reach those goals, lead to actions. Actions lead to tangible results, and results lead to the body, life, and purpose you want to achieve.

Confusion, on the other hand, overwhelms you, leading to frustration, paralysis, and that dead-end situation where you're eating exactly the way you've always eaten just because it's easier. And, of course, if you end up doing what you've always done, you'll get the same results you've always gotten. You'll feel trapped in that downward spiral of feeling badly about how you look and feel.

But you are *not* going to that desperate place again! Look at how far you've come, my friend. Learning, opening doors of awareness, and following that inner voice that demands the best are more than half the battle. Clear your head, visualize the direction you want to go, and keep putting one of those lovely feet in front of the other. Remember, the only slip up is to give up. And this much I know – you are not going to give up. You must keep building that one and only house in which you reside lifelong – your body.

I suggest that you read and refer to these chapters over and over again. Nothing can replace studying, time, effort, and lots of repetition. You will find that the information in this book will be a valuable tool for building a rock-solid foundation of basic food and health facts that will help guide you as you learn more. Here are some key points to take with you:

1. **Ignore and dismiss myths, misconceptions, half-truths, or whole lies** that bombard you every day from the media, doctors, authors, talk-show gurus, well-intended, but sabotaging family and friends, and your own self-talk. Write

down the sound bites of information and actually compare it to the facts in this book, as well as others you find as you (hopefully) read even more about the ideas in 10+10. When you hear these sound bites, ask yourself, "Does this make sense?" Trust *your* guts.

2. <u>**Learn and live by nature's simple principle**</u>: whole, fresh fruits and vegetables are your weight warriors and health heroes. They are full of all the macro nutrients (proteins, carbohydrates, and fats), vitamins, minerals, enzymes, fiber, and micronutrients necessary for building health and shedding fat.

3. <u>**Lose weight and keep weight off forever**</u> by following the three 10+10 rules: Add, Stop, and Wiggle (if you must!). Fill up on the feed-me, best-for-you foods first, stop eating when you're full, and wiggle when you absolutely have to – but *no more* than 20% of the time, and less if you want to lose more weight, more quickly.

4. <u>**Build an arsenal of simple, logical answers to the four most common questions**</u> to reinforce your knowledge and to build your confidence with the facts.

   a. If I don't eat meat, where do I get my protein?

   b. If I don't eat dairy, where do I get my calcium?

   c. But don't carbs make me fat?

   d. But isn't olive oil a good fat?

Stop listening to hearsay, no matter what bull, with or without credentials, is charging you. Learn the facts about feeding and depleting foods (Chapter 5), proteins (Chapter 11), good and bad carbs (Chapter

12), good and bad fats (chapter 13), and dairy/calcium (Chapter 14). And, after you get a handle on these facts, read as many other credible sources as you can to reinforce this knowledge. And, by credible, I don't mean the news media. Read health journals and magazines. Look up studies on the Internet. Read some of the books I've referenced and some of the books those books reference.

With practice, you will know the health facts cold, and you will feel comfortable when someone challenges your way of eating because you will have an arsenal of real facts, real studies, and fact-based knowledge. However, until you get a good handle on things and feel really comfortable, I would deflect these challenges and questions. Don't let anyone change your mind. If the person really knows the facts and has an open mind, he or she will whole-heartedly agree with you instead of defending his or her bad habits.

Or, you can answer challenging questions by falling back on this book with this very simple, genuine, and kind response: "Dr. Leslie answers that question and discusses that issue in *Getting Into Your Pants*. Why don't you read it, and then let's have a conversation about it when you're done. That will help me understand it better myself."

Most people won't bother reading. And, if they don't, don't waste your time with them and don't allow yourself to get dragged into a discussion based on emotion and ignorance. Your time and energy are worth too much to waste. Besides, negativity is dangerously sabotaging and contagious. Get good at calmly stepping out of the way, allowing those bulls to charge right past you.

With humility, stand quietly strong and confident with what you know to be true. Know that you are different and know that you've got to be different to make a difference in your life and the lives of others.

Losing weight is not just about slimming down – it's about shedding layers, lasering into your core, building self-esteem, and evolving into all that you are. It's about the freedom to be you and all that you were born to be. As my dear friend and mentor, Dr. Tony Palermo, says, it's about calling forth your greatness. Go forward and call forth your greatness because you are beyond great – you are extraordinary.

And when you do get scoffed at and riveted with questions from people who don't have your knowledge, your insights, and your guts to follow-through – and mark my words, you will – be amused by our own, private, little joke. "Ahhh, Dr. Leslie told me I would be asked that." Just giggle quietly to yourself and stay on track to lose that jiggle. Above all else, we must have giggles along the way, especially about our own wiggles and jiggles.

5. **When you get to that magical moment – you watch, about 15 or 20 pounds down – when that first person asks you this question, "How did you lose all that weight?" answer like this with graciousness and gratitude:** "I am simply eating better by filling up on more fruits and vegetables. It works for me." Don't justify. Don't judge. Don't preach. And learn to duck. It's not about being right – it's about doing what's *right* for you.

Now go for it! Do what's right for you. Take the information that you have worked so hard to learn and start building yourself that dream house in which you live – your body – for life. Feed it. Move it. Nurture it. Appreciate it. Treasure it. Love it. Honor it. And by all means, grace it with those pants – *your* pants.

WHAT YOU NOW KNOW...

- How to create a doable, yearlong, weight-loss plan-of-action.

- How to choose and track monthly action steps to reach your one-year goals.

- How to simplify 10+10 food shopping and organize your kitchen.

- How to prepare one week of 10+10 meals.

- How to shed layers, inside and out, and do what's right for you to build your dream house – your body and your life, for life.

Feed-Me Food-for-Thought

"You are the master of your own choices and either the beneficiary of or slave to the consequences."

– Dr. Leslie Van Romer

INSPIRATIONAL

- You've got to be different to make a difference.

- Be the hero of your body-dream-come-true.

- It's not about being right; it's about doing what's right for you.

- You deserve to feel good about you.

- Body first; everything else second.

- Success is getting up one more time than you fall.

- The only slip up is to give up.

- The tough right choice today is much easier than no choice tomorrow.

- You got to be selfish to be self-less.

- Your outer world is the exact reflection of your inner world.

- She was the richest woman in the graveyard, so what? Wealth can't buy health.

- When a bull comes charging at you, step out of the way.

- The you tomorrow is worth your effort today.

- Clear intentions will attract the right people, support, and material assistance needed for your solo, noble journey to the best you.

- Trust yourself, don't tempt yourself.

GETTING INTO YOUR PANTS

- Fat – the silent enemy that maims and kills.

- Genetics load the gun, you pull the trigger.

- You were birthed from the loins of our culture; our culture created food monsters.

- You didn't have a fighting chance since birth; you do now.

- You are no more weak, lazy, undisciplined than the rest of us mere mortals – you're simply a product of your conditioning.

- Food: our greatest comfort, our greatest pain.

- The label you give yourself is not important; what you feed yourself is.

- You didn't fail; the diets failed you.

- To get into your pants, you've got to really want it.

- To lose weight, reconnect the disconnect between you and food.

- Shifting is the key to losing weight: shift thinking, choices, habits, and lifestyle.

- To subtract weight, think addition, not subtraction, deprivation, starving, and guilting.

- Fruits and vegetables give you the most nutrition for your calorie buck.

- Does this food feed me or deplete me?

- Fill up on the best-for-you foods first.

- Eat the good guys first and the bad guys last.

- Fruits and vegetables – weight and disease warriors and energy and health heroes.

- 10+10 for Life® = 10 fruits and 10 vegetables a day, every day.

- The three 10+10 rules for weight loss and body-best: Add, Stop, and Wiggle (if you must!)

- Fruits are the fastest fast foods: wash, open mouth, insert, and chew.

- Eating vegetables is like eating air – very few calories.

- Your energy today is sourced by the good carbs – fruits and vegetables – you ate yesterday.

- Proteins build your engine; carbohydrates provide the fuel to make your engine run.

- With time and patience, the effort-full evolves into effort-less.

- Extra cals are not your pals, gals.

- Fat goes from your lips to your hips so get a grip.

- The fat you eat is the fat you wear, the same fat that maims and kills.

- Extra fat is bad fat whether it comes from a cow, chicken, fish, or olive.

- Olive oil is good for two things: more calories and more fat.

- Only people milk is perfect for baby people.

- Garbage disposals are replaceable; you are not.

- Raw is better than cooked, plant is better than animal, and no added oils – period!

- If it has a label, don't buy it.

- It's not about self-control; it's about auto-stop by filling up on the best-for-you foods first.

- If you won't make wiser choices for you, do it for those who love and need you.

- Do elephants eat hamburgers, chicken, fish, tofu, or protein bars to get protein for their great, big muscles? No, they eat whole plant foods.

- Do cows drink milk and eat cheese to get their calcium for big, strong bones and teeth and milk in their udders? No, they eat whole plant foods.

- Meat and dairy are choices with consequences, not necessities.

- Exercise doesn't take time, it gives you time when it counts – at the end of your life.

- Getting weight loss advice from someone overweight and unfit is like getting financial advice from a guy driving a broken down Pinto.

- You've got nothing to lose – except weight – and everything to gain – like life.

- The body you want is waiting, so what big but is stopping you?

- If you have the want, the will, and the direction, you will find your way.

- Wiggle a little to lose that jiggle.

Sources

"Losing weight is a shedding process – from the inside out."

– Dr. Leslie Van Romer

Chapter 2

Bowman SA, Gormaker SL, Ebbeling CB, Pereira MA, Ludwig DS. "Effects of fast food consumption on energy intake and diet quality among children in a national household survey." *Pediatrics,* 113: 112-118, 2004.

Campbell, T. Colin. *The China Study.* Dallas: BenBella, 2005.

Colditz, et al, "Weight as a Risk Factor for Clinical Diabetes in Women," *American Journal of Epidemiology,* 132: 501-513, 1990.

Fuhrman, Joel. *Eat to Live.* Boston: Little, Brown and Company, 2003.

Greg, Critser. *Fat Land: How Americans Became the Fattest People in the World.* Boston: Houghton Mifflin Company, 2003.

Newman, Cathy. "Why Are We So Fat?," *National Geographic,* 46, Aug. 2004.

"Overweight, Obesity and Health Risk." *Archives of Internal Medicine.* National Task Force on the Prevention and Treatment of Obesity, 160: 898-904, 2000.

"Prevalence of Overweight and Obesity Among Adults: United States, 2003-2004." *National Center for Health Statistics.*

Robbins, John. *Food Revolution.* Berkeley: Conari Press, 2001.

Root, Mary, "Obesity and Health: A Hard Look at the Data." *Our Food Our Future.* New Century Nutrition: Earthsave International, 2007.

Schlosser, Eric. *Fast Food Nation.* Boston: Houghton Mifflin Company, 2005.

Wyatt, C., et al, "Dietary Intake of Sodium, Potassium, and Blood Pressure in Lacto-Ovo Vegetarians," *Nutrition Research,* 15:819-830, 1995.

Chapter 3

Fuhrman, Joel. Eat to Live. Boston: Little, Brown and Company, 2003.

Chapter 6

Diamond, Harvey and Marilyn. Fit for Life. New York: Warner Books, 1985.

Chapter 9

Albertson, Ellen, "Wake Up – Without Caffeine." Natural Health, Jan/Feb 1995.

American Diabetes Association's 64th Scientific Sessions, Orlando, Fla., June 4-8. News release, American Diabetes Association, 2004.

Appleton, Nancy. Lick the Sugar Habit. U.S.A.: Avery, 1996.

Barnard, Neal. Breaking the Food Seduction. New York: St. Martin's, 2004.

Barnard, Neal, et al. Nutrition Guide for Clinicians. Washington, D.C.: 1st ed. Physician's Committee for Responsible Medicine, 2007.

Davis, Brenda. Melina, Vesanto. Becoming Vegan. Summertown, Tennessee: Book Publishing Company, 2000.

Dhingra, Ravi. MD, et al. "Soft Drink Consumption and Risk of Developing Cardiometabolic Risk Factors and the Metabolic Syndrome in Middle-Aged Adults in the Community." Circulation, 116: 480-8, Jul 2007.

Fuhrman, Joel. Eat to Live. Boston: Little, Brown, and Company, 2001.

Novick, Jeff. "Waking Up to the Effects of Caffeine." Health Science. Spring 2002.

Robbins, John. The Food Revolution. Berkeley: Conari Press, 2001.

Roberts, H. J. "Townsend Letter for Doctors and Patients." Jan 2000.

Chapter 10

Barnard, Neal, et al. Nutrition Guide for Clinicians. Washington, D.C.: 1st ed. Physician's Committee for Responsible Medicine, 2007.

Campbell, T. Colin. The China Study. Dallas: BenBella, 2005.

Davis, Brenda. Melina, Vesanto. Becoming Vegan. Summertown, Tennessee: Book

Publishing Company, 2000.

Diamond, Harvey, and Marilyn Diamond. *Fit for Life*. New York: Warner Books, 1985.

McDougall, John. *The McDougall Program – 12 Days to Dynamic Health*. New York: Penguin Group, 1991.

Morck, T. "Inhibition of Food Iron Absorption by Coffee." American Journal of Clinical Nutrition, 37: 416, 1983.

Quigley, EM, Carmichael, HA, Watkinson, G. "Adult celiac disease (celiac sprue), pernicious anemia and IgA deficiency: case report and review of the relationships between Vitamin B12 deficiency, small intestinal mucosal disease and immunoglobulin deficiency." *Journal of Clinical Gastroenterology*, 8:277-281, 1983.

Chapter 11

Barnard, Neal D., et al. *Nutrition Guide for Clinicians*, 1st ed. Physician's Committee for Responsible Medicine, 2007.

Campbell, T. Colin. *The China Study*. Dallas: BenBella Books, 2005.

Havala, S. and Dwyer, J. "Position of the American Dietetic Association: vegetarian diets-technical support paper." *Journal American Dietetics Association*, 88: 352-5, 1988.

McDougall, John. *The McDougall Program – 12 Days to Dynamic Health*. New York: Penguin Group, 1991.

Robbins, John. *Diet for a New America*. Walpole: Stillpoint Publishing, 1987.

Chapter 12

Appleton, Nancy. *Lick the Sugar Habit*. U.S.A.: Avery, 1996.

Barnard, Neal. *Breaking the Food Seduction*. New York: St. Martin's, 2004.

Barnard, Neal, et al. *Nutrition Guide for Clinicians*. Washington, D.C.: 1st ed. Physician's Committee for Responsible Medicine, 2007.

Davis, Brenda. Melina, Vesanto. *Becoming Vegan*. Summertown, Tennessee: Book Company, 2000.

Fuhrman, Joel. *Eat to Live*. Boston: Little, Brown, and Company, 2001.

McDougall, John, M.D., *The McDougall Program, 12 Days to Dynamic Health*. New York: Penguin Group, 1990.

Chapter 13

Campbell, Colin T. *The China Study*. Dallas: BenBella, 2005.

Esselstyn, Caldwell B. *Prevent and Reverse Heart Disease*, U.S.A.: Avery, 2007.

Fuhrman, Joel. *Eat to Live*. Boston: Little, Brown, and Company, 2001.

McDougall, John. *The McDougall Program for a Healthy Heart*. New York: Penguin Group,1996.

Pizzorno, Joseph E., Michael T. Murray, and Churchill Livingstone. *Textbook of Natural Medicine*, V1-140: 172, 1999.

Willett, WC, MJ Stampfer, JE Manson, GA Colditz, FE Speizer, BA Rosner, LA Sampson, CH Hennekens. "Intake of Trans Fatty Acids and Risk of Coronary Heart Disease among Women." *Lancet*, 341:581-585, Mar 1993.

Chapter 14

Calkins, B., et al. "Diet Nutrition Intake and Metabolism in Populations." *Journal of the American Dietetic Association*, 77: 655-661, 1980.

Campbell, Colin T. *The China Study*. Summertown, Tennessee: BenBella, 2005.

Chan, J.M., Giovannucci, E.L. "Dairy products, calcium, and vitamin D and risk of prostate cancer." *Epidemiology Revs*, 23:87-92, 2001.

Chen, H., O'Reilly, E. McCullough, M.L., Rodriguez, C., et al. "Consumption of Dairy Products and Risk of Parkinson's Disease." *American Journal of Epidemiology*, 165:998-1006, 2007.

Cramer, D.W., Harlow, B.L., Willet, W.C. "Galactose consumption and metabolism in relation to the risk of ovarian cancer." *Lancet*, 2: 66-71, 1989.

Donham, K.J. "Epidemiologic relationships of the bovine population and human leukemia in Iowa." *American Journal of Epidemiology*, 112(1):80-92, July 1980.

Fuhrman, Joel. *Eat to Live*. Boston: Little, Brown and Company, 2003.

Gordon, T, WP Castelli, MC Hjortland, et al, "Predicting coronary heart disease in middle-aged and older person," The Framingham study. *Journal of American Medical Association*, 238(6):497-499, Aug 1977.

Holmes, M.D. "Dietary correlates of plasma insulin-like growth factor 1 and insulin-like growth factor binding protein 3 concentrations." *Cancer Epidemiologic Biomarkers Prevention*, 9:852-61, Sep 11, 2002.

Howell, M.A. "Factor analysis of international cancer mortality data and per capita food consumption." *British Journal of Cancer*, 4:328-36, Apr 29, 1974.

Hursting, S.D. "Diet and human leukemia: an analysis of international data." *Preventative Medicine*, 3:409-22, May 22, 1993.

Iacono, G. "Intolerance of cow's milk and chronic constipation in children." *North England Journal of Medicine*, 339(15):1100-1104. Oct 1998.

"Infant feeding practices and their possible relationship to the etiology of diabetes mellitus." *Pediatrics*, Work Group on Cow's Milk Protein and Diabetes Mellitus, 1994.

Juntti, H. "Cow's milk allergy is associated with recurrent otitis media during childhood." *Acta Oto-Laryngologica*, 119(8): 867-73, 1999.

Kradjian, Robert M. "The Milk Letter." *Earthsave*, 2002.

McDougall, John. "Dairy Products and 10 False Promises." *The McDougall Newsletter 2*, 2003.

McDougall, John. "Marketing Milk and Disease." *The McDougall Newsletter 2*, 2003.

McDougall, John. *The McDougall Program for a Healthy Heart*. New York: Penguin Group, 1996.

Mead, Nathanial. "Don't Drink Your Milk." *Health Freedom News*, 37, March 1995.

Mepham, T.B. "Safety of milk from cows treated with bovine somatotropin." *Lancet*, 44 (8916):197-8, July 3, 1994.

Mettlin, C.J., Piver, M.S. "A case-control study of milk-drinking and ovarian cancer risk." *American Journal of Epidemiology*, 132 (5):871-876, 1990.

Robbins, John. *The Food Revolution*. Berkeley: Conari Press, 2001.

Yimyaem, P. "Gastrointestinal manifestations of Cow's milk protein allergy during the first year of life." *Journal Medical Association of Thailand*, 86(2): 116-23, Feb, 2003.

Yu, H. "Role of the insulin-like growth factor family in cancer development and progression." *Journal National Cancer Institute*, 92(18): 1472-1489, Sep 20, 2000.

Index

Meet the Author

D r. Leslie Van Romer received her Bachelor of Science from the State University of New York at Cortland and her Doctor of Chiropractic from Sherman College of Straight Chiropractic in South Carolina, where she graduated as summa cum laude and class valedictorian.

Since then, she has spent close to thirty years building a thriving, full-time practice and developing a wide variety of motivational health presentations, along with accompanying DVDs and CDs. Dr. Leslie created her own registered weight-loss, body-best program, called 10+10 for Life®, and writes *Dr. Leslie's Lifelines*, a free weekly online newsletter.

Motivated by the desire for better health and ideal weight for herself and her family, Dr. Leslie early on began to look into the root cause of the overweight epidemic and the diseases which disable and kill most Americans – the American diet, with its heavy emphasis on high-fat, high-cholesterol, high-animal protein, high-chemical, and high-calorie foods. The more she studied, the more she became aware and appalled that theories behind our focus on meat and dairy products were not only flawed, but dangerous, and that our eating habits had been further skewed by pressure from the food industry and our own ignorance, confusion, and spoiled taste buds.

Further inspired by her own daughter's struggle with weight, Dr. Leslie not only adopted a truly nutritionally sound, plant-based diet for herself and her children, but she naturally gravitated toward helping her patients lose weight and build health. Dr. Leslie's weight-loss program evolved from her cumulative years of research, experience, and just good ole' common sense. 10+10 for Life® offers hope, simple direction, and ongoing support. Dr. Leslie's passion for people and her life's mission make her and her dedicated team very accessible and approachable.

Dr. Leslie has expertly helped thousands of people sort fact from fiction, shift their eating and lifestyle choices, and shed the layers, inside and out. She lives her talk and leads by example. By following 10+10 for Life® for years and exercising at least an hour a day, Dr. Leslie maintains her ideal weight and level of energy, fitness, and health.

Dr. Leslie authored the 8-day, on-line course, *The Body You Want Wants You Too – Say Goodbye to Yo-Yo Diets and Lose Weight-Forever,* and wrote and produced *A Journey to a Whole New You,* a 6-CD audio series, featuring *Kiss Yo-Yo Diets Goodbye – Forever.* She has written well over 100 weight-loss and health-related articles.

As a single mom, Dr. Leslie raised three children in the foothills of the Olympic Mountains in the lovely town of Sequim, WA. They are now young adults and successfully finding their own paths.

Attend Dr. Leslie's Pants Party by Phone

I am throwing a Pants Party, and **you are invited** to come and join in the fun – free of charge! Just send your name and email address to **info@drleslievanromer.com** and put "Pants Party" in the subject line. You will receive the date of the party, your pass code, and directions to the Pants Party by Phone in plenty of time before the date.

During the first telephone Pants Party by Phone, you will learn:

1. How to lose weight – permanently – by following just three easy 10+10 rules: Add, Stop, and Wiggle (if you must).

2. How to cheat – guilt-free.

3. How to crush cravings.

4. How to tell the difference between feed-me vs. deplete-me foods.

5. How to stay full and satisfied and still lose weight, without depriving, starving, counting, measuring, fussing, or guilting ever again.

6. How to form a reasonable, yearlong, weight-loss goal.

7. How to stay on track with 5 doable monthly action steps.

8. How to plan breakfast, lunch, dinner, and snacks.

9. How to make you and your family happy with one meal.

10. How to feel good about YOU every step of the way.

Join me and meet others just like you for the fun, facts, and most importantly of all, renewed self-confidence and hope that you can get into those pants – one bite at a time.

Email today to get on our list. We will contact you with the Pants Party by Phone details.

Quick Order Form

Fax orders: 360-683-5381. Send this form.

Telephone orders: Call 360-683-8844 or 1-888-drleslie (888-375-3754). Have your credit card ready.

Email orders: info@drlesievanromer.com

Postal Orders: Dr. Leslie Van Romer, 415 North Sequim Ave, Sequim, WA 98382

_____**Please send me (**_____**) copies of** *Getting Into Your Pants* **at $18.99 per book plus tax of 8.4% (only if shipped to Washington State address) and (**_____**) shipping as stated below.**

GRAND TOTAL: $_____

_____**I'm emailing my email address to** info@drlesievanromer.com **and putting "e-letter" in subject to receive my FREE Dr. Leslie's Lifelines. (Look in websites** www.gettingintoyourpants.com **and** www.drlesievanromer.com **for information, articles, products, and services.)**

_____**I'm interested in Dr. Leslie's Pants Party by Phone, my first one FREE of charge to me if I enroll now by emailing in my registration with "Pants Party" in the subject line. Offer good until March 1, 2009.**

_____**I'm interested in submitting my personal Pants Story to be included in the follow-up Advanced Pants book for the grand prize of four personal coaching sessions with Dr. Leslie herself (a $1000.00 value). Email me with the information.**

Name: _____

Address: _____

City: _____**State:**_____**Zip:**_____

Telephone: _____

Email address: _____

Sales Tax: Please add 8.4% sales tax for products shipped to Washington State addresses.

Handling and shipping:

U.S.: $4.00 for first book or disk, $2.00 for each additional item

International: $9.00 for first book or disk; $5.00 for each additional item

Payment: ____Check ____Credit Card: ____Visa ____ MasterCard

Card number: _____

Name on card: _____Exp. Date: _____

Order the Tools to Help You Get Into Your Pants

If you desire every opportunity to get into your pants and stay in them, consider giving your-self one or both of these invaluable tools: The *Getting Into Your Pants PlayBook*, your chapter-by-chapter companion guide (workbook) to Getting Into Your Pants – lickety split, and the *Pants Weight-Loss Pocket Calendar* to help formulate and record personal yearlong goals and monthly action steps, as well as track all the things you did right for one year.

Fax orders: 360-683-5381. Send this form.

Telephone orders: Call 360-683-8844 or 1-888-drleslie (888-375-3754). Have your credit card ready.

Email orders: info@drleslievanromer.com

Postal Orders: Dr. Leslie Van Romer, 415 North Sequim Ave, Sequim, WA 98382

_____Please send me (_____) copies of *Getting Into Your Pants* at $18.99 per book plus tax of 8.4% (only if shipped to Washington State address) and (_____) shipping as stated below.

GRAND TOTAL: $_____

_____Please send me (_____) copies of the *Pants PlayBook* at $10.99 per book plus tax of 8.4% (only if shipped to Washington State address) and (_____) shipping as stated below.

GRAND TOTAL: $_____

_____Please send me (_____) copies of the *Pants Weight-Loss Pocket Calendar* at $7.95 per cal-endar plus tax of 8.4% (only if shipped to Washington State address) and free shipping.

GRAND TOTAL: $_____

Name: _____

Address: _____

City: _____State:_____Zip:_____

Telephone: _____

Email address: _____

Sales Tax: Please add 8.4% sales tax for products shipped to Washington State addresses.

Handling and shipping: U.S.: $4.00 for first book, $2.00 for each additional item

International: $9.00 for first book; $5.00 for each additional item

Payment: ___Check   ___Credit Card: ___Visa ___ MasterCard

Card number: _____

Name on card: _____Exp. Date: _____